For Only One Day

How focusing on one action, for one day, can change your life.

By Sonia Goforth

Pendem Publishing, LLC

For Only One Day

How focusing on one action, for one day, can change your life

ISBN: 978-0-9972242-0-7

Library of Congress Control Number: 2016931165

Published by Pendem Publishing, LLC

1050 Buckley Ln

Lawrenceburg, KY 40342

http://pendempub.com

Edited by Jamie Ogles

Cover design by timrevel.com

Dedication

This book is dedicated to my grandson, Eli.

In Heaven, I hope you know how much you meant to us, and changed our lives, in the short time you were here.

Acknowledgements

I would first like to thank my husband, Ed, who supports me through every crazy idea, and has even suggested a few of his own. In you, I have a spouse and a best friend. I can't imagine spending the rest of this insane life with anyone else.

Thank you to my family. Every single one of you thought this book was a great idea and supported me completely. Words won't express how much you mean to me. We've shared so much together, and whether good or bad, we just seem to grow closer.

Thank you to my editor, Jamie. You epitomize how an editorial relationship should be. Guiding me through the process, you challenged me to pull out more and become a better writer. I consider you a dear friend, and I hope to work many more years together.

Thank you to Peggy DeKay, book coach. The chat we had during the lunch break at the Carnegie Literary Conference proved to be one of the best hours of my literary journey to date. Your advice impacted me, and your book helped me find my way through the dark.

To the members of the Badass Girls Club, Amanda, EB, Dani, Tammy & Caroline, thank you for your never ending support and love. Thank you for pushing me to do this, and giving me a cheering section along the way. We *can* make our dreams happen!

To my long-time friend Kathryn, thank you for being my spiritual support and personal cheerleader. The long talks we've had about life and paths have meant more than you will ever know. You're one of my dearest friends, and I hope to repay you one day with the support you've given me.

To Hannah and the employees at the Jessamine Co. Starbucks, thank you for letting me have a quiet spot to work and words of encouragement. It's nice to have a home away from home.

The same thank you goes to the staff at the Jessamine County Library. A smiling face on the way in and a table to write at was just what I needed to keep me moving forward.

Contents

Introduction

He weighed 1.5lbs.

He was the most precious thing I had ever seen.

I was honored to be one of the ones holding and loving him as he took his last breaths.

Life can be cruelly beautiful!

My grandson, Eli, was born at 24 weeks and weighed 1.9lbs. He was a tiny miracle and a fighter from the start. Unfortunately, the fight was more than his little body could handle, and eleven days later, he was gone.

There are moments in your life that cut you open, leave you bleeding and, if you survive, provide scars you'll carry for the rest of your life. There are other moments that have you soaring with joy higher than the clouds above Mt. Olympus. When Eli came into our world, we experienced both.

Eli's birth and passing came at the tail end of a period in my family's history that forever changed our definition of normal. We had unexpectedly lost five family members in the four years prior to his arrival. It already felt as if God had it in for us, and taking Eli was the final blow. Once again, we stood at a funeral absolutely numb and going through motions we knew all too well. It wasn't enough to lose my grandmother, sister-in-law, father-in-law, brother-in-law, and cousin. We had yet one more obstacle to overcome.

I don't know if it's from strength, fear, or just being so worn down we don't know what else to do, but we're surviving as a family and we're closer than we've ever been. It hasn't been easy. My husband is my mother-in-law's only surviving child. We now find ourselves the matriarch and patriarch to a family dealing with great loss. My Christmas stocking count has gone from five to twenty-two. It's been a crazy ride, and I think we're all dealing with a little bit of PTSD.

It's also been an incredible ride of self-discovery. You never know what you're capable of until circumstances force you to be and do more than you ever thought you could. That's where this book came from. I'm not a doctor or psychiatrist. I have no degrees in social work or counseling. The closest I've ever come to those are my college psychology courses or my years in personal therapy. Everything I've learned has been hands-on, pick-yourself-off-the-ground-and-dust-yourself-off lessons.

It was after Eli that I began actually doing small things to make myself feel better. I was tired of feeling down. I was tired of reading and hearing self-help theory. I wanted actual results. I wanted to feel whole again, or as close to whole as I could possibly get. This is where *For Only One Day* got its start. I thought if I could concentrate on one thing each day--because that's all I had the energy for--maybe it would make a difference over time.

It did, and I felt a slow semblance of the person I once was begin to reappear.

I started playing with the things I would work on each day. I took all the theory and ideas from the different books I was reading and created actions I could focus on. I began having fun with it, and what developed has become a standard for the way I now try to live.

This book is all about actions. *Physically* doing things each day. You can have all the theory in the world, but if it never culminates into action, it's never going to do you any good. In the following pages, you'll find ninety different actions. Pick one each day to focus on. I don't care if you go in order or if you choose which one to do each day or if you just randomly open the book and let fate decide for you; the important thing is that you *do* them. Give them a try. If you like what you focused on, then keep doing it. If you didn't, then you haven't wasted a lot of time and you can move onto something new tomorrow. The thing is, you *tried* it. At the end of each day, take a moment and look at the questions under Refection Time. These can help you digest what you learned through the day.

I truly believe that these actions are what saved my sanity and are helping me move forward in my life. I won't promise results of wine and roses, but these actions can make things a bit better instead of just wishing. My hope is that by sharing these, I can help others make improvements in their lives. It may be bit by bit, but it's a start.

I believe we are all here on this earth for a purpose. I don't know exactly what Eli's was, but I would bet it was to make a difference in all the lives he touched. If that's the case, he succeeded brilliantly. My goal is to have the lessons he taught me reach others. Life is meant to be lived. I guess that's the greatest lesson I've learned from everyone my family has lost.

May you always see the road ahead with light instead of darkness.

Sonia

No judgement

The guy driving too close to our bumper is an ass, the crazy lady behind us in the checkout line is on something, and the woman with the screaming kid at the grocery store is a bad parent and needs to discipline her child. Face it; we judge all day long.

Is it possible to stop judging altogether? In 2014, a study in the *Journal of Neuroscience* done by researchers at Dartmouth College showed that our brains work so fast that they will judge a person's face as trustworthy or not trustworthy before the face is even fully perceived.[1] So

[1] Jonathan B. Freeman, et all. "Amygdala Responsivity to High-Level Social Information from Unseen Faces" . *The Journal of Neuroscience*. 6 August 2014. http://psych.nyu.edu/freemanlab/pubs/2014Freeman_JNeuro.pd

while we apparently are hardwired to make judgements extremely fast, we need to slow it down a bit.

The first step is to notice when you're judging. You may not realize how much you make judgements until you become aware by monitoring your thoughts.

The reality is, we can let the guy riding our bumper pass and he can be an ass to someone else. Hopefully, karma will intervene and we'll pass him later as he's getting a ticket from the boys in blue. Anyone who's had kids can sympathize with needing a gallon of milk and having your three-year-old throw a tantrum of epic proportions because you won't buy them the package of pure sugar conveniently stocked next to them in the checkout isle. The crazy lady behind us? Well, unless she's your mother, you probably won't have to see her again, so life is okay.

<u>Today's Action:</u>

Focus energy on your own productivity instead of what's around you. Try not to judge anything, and if you find yourself jumping to judgement, shift your focus somewhere else. If you need to wear a rubber band around your wrist and snap it each time you catch yourself, beautiful! When I did this, it was incredibly refreshing to let things around me simply exist. I didn't have to expend mental energy bringing any more drama into my head. I also quickly discovered that the skin on the inside of the wrist is particularly sensitive to pain.

Reflection Time:

- How did going through a day and not making judgements make you feel?
- How was your day better by doing this?
- How could you implement this into your everyday?
- How shocked were you at how often you had to correct yourself?

Car Dance

What do you do when you desperately want to sing at the top of your lungs to Dancing Queen by ABBA but you're afraid you'll look like an idiot to the people in the cars around you?

You do it!

You don't know those other people and, even if you did, so what? Truth be known, some of them secretly wish they had your guts. The others, who also enjoy taking a few minutes and releasing from society's norms, may reciprocate and start their own dance party.

Ignore the etiquette instructions you received as a child on what is the "appropriate" way to act in public.

Those lessons were for your parent's benefit, not yours. Can you help it if they were mortified when you stripped naked and ran around the toy store hooting like a Native American ready for a buffalo hunt? It certainly wasn't your fault that the President of the Women's League was two isles over.

Today's Action:

We let other's opinions of us carry too much weight. When one of your favorite songs comes on the radio today, car dance! I don't care who's in the lane next to you. Free yourself for a whole 3 minutes and see what happens. I can just about guarantee you'll start laughing and feel wonderful!

Now, for those of you who've never car danced, it's really easy. Start small, maybe with tapping on the steering wheel. Then move to bobbing the head. Start by mouthing the words or singing in a light voice. As you get more comfortable, escalate the tone and increase the head bobbing. Swing the shoulders side to side and, before you know it, you're CAR DANCING!

Now, for safety reasons, if you're going to do any serious head banging, stretch first. My husband threw down to Van Halen's *Hot for Teacher* and actually pulled a muscle. Thank goodness *he* was driving, because I almost peed my pants laughing. Also, if you have teenagers, this is a great way to totally embarrass them. My son, to this day, will tell you about the time the officer saw me car dancing. I'm having a great time, the officer's smirking trying to hold it together, and my son is in the floor dying. It was terrific!

Reflection Time:

- How did letting yourself go for three minutes make you feel?
- Why do you think you were self-conscious, if you were?
- What are three songs you're definitely going to need to car dance to?

Grateful List

We are all grateful for things – our family, our friends, our health and the lady at the drive-thru handing out double quarter pounders on those *really* bad days! But have we taken the time to list them all on a piece of paper to get it out of our heads?

Dr. Emmons and Dr. McCullough, psychologists with the University of California and the University of Miami, presented a study showing how writing about things you are grateful for each week for a 10-week period can actually increase optimism and positive feelings about life.[2] It's just really hard to think about how grateful you

---

[2] Emmons RA, et al. "Counting Blessings Versus Burdens: An Experimental Investigation of Gratitude and Subjective Well-Being in Daily Life," *Journal of*

are for the beautiful sunny day when the white car with the bitchy lady just stole the parking spot you've been trying to get for ten minutes. Now, you're going to have to park in the back forty and hoof across a football field to pick up the specific *Paw Patrol* doll your nephew wants for his birthday and can apparently only be found in this one store. You're just grateful you don't strangle her at the cart stall.

Today's Action:

Sit down with a piece of paper and do a mind dump of everything and anything you are grateful for. It doesn't matter how small or crazy. For example: I'm grateful for my family and I'm also grateful that every other Friday I sleep with an octopus - aka my grandson - who leaves me with two inches of bed up against a wall. I wouldn't trade it for the world even though I wake up immediately needing an appointment with my chiropractor.

When you're done, look over and really notice all in your life you are thankful for. I was blown away the first

---

Personality and Social Psychology(Feb. 2003): Vol. 84, No. 2, pp. 377–89.

time I did this. Looking at all the good in my life made the bad less noticeable and easier to dismiss. Now, every evening I list five things I was grateful for that day. Some regular candidates are my husband, my sanity, and the bag of chocolate in my bottom dresser drawer.

Reflection Time:

- What did it feel like to list and focus on all the good in your life instead of all the bad?
- What revelations did you come up with in doing this?
- What are some of the things you are regularly grateful for?

Speed Limit

Okay, you're probably saying to yourself, "You've got to be crazy telling me that driving the speed limit can help me create a better life!"

First, let's look at the way most of us usually drive. You get in your car on your way to work. You crank up the radio's volume, coffee positioned at three o'clock, a quick self-check in the mirror, and you're prepared for battle. Muscles are tense and ready, we've practiced our scowl and we've become skilled at the sign language of telling people they are number one. Now, it's just a matter of getting out there and trying to go as fast as we can without attracting undue attention causing those flashing blue lights to appear behind us. Our bumper sticker proudly states "I may be slow but at least I'm in front of you!"

What are we *doing*? We're tense and anxious before we even leave the driveway! I've actually caught myself gritting my teeth so hard my jaw begins to ache. SLOW DOWN! It's not a race for your life!

Lifehacker actually shows where, mathematically, speeding only helps on really long car trips and almost all theoretical gains are lost in traffic due to any number of things.[3] So why do we continue to create stress for ourselves just by sitting in our car?

Today's Action:

Take the day and go the speed limit. For some, this will be agonizing as you watch cars pass. Resist the temptation to join the Indy 500. Breathe! It will be ok. I promise you won't spontaneously combust if you don't

---

[3] Ravenscraft, Eric. "Does Speeding Really Get You There Any Faster?" Lifehacker.com. http://lifehacker.com/does-speeding-really-get-you-there-any-faster-1556767685. (accessed January 4, 2016)

prove your Corolla can outrun the Porsche. Let others pass in stress-mode. Listen to your favorite music. Sing! Car dance! Enjoy the trip! This isn't your personal version of an illegal street race.

Your body, your car and your wallet will thank you.

Reflection Time:

- How did it feel to go against the norm and slow down for the day?
- If it was unnerving at first, how were you able to get past it and go with the flow?
- How did you notice your body position and breath changing during this action versus how it usually is?

Damn, You're Good-Looking

I've always been jealous that no matter the version of the Snow White story, each time The Evil Queen looks into her mirror to ask the infamous question, she looks immaculate. Do you think she looks like that right out of bed or is always looking fabulous a perk of having evil magical powers?

Apparently I missed the day when they were handing out these powers because that's definitely not me! Each morning, my hair looks like a couple of field rats nested in it for the winter, I have two black eyes from the mascara I forgot to take off, and, depending on how hard I slept, I may have a line of dried drool going from the corner of my mouth around my chin and down my neck. I couldn't look into any mirror and ask that question with a straight face.

But why is that? Why can't I look into the mirror and say "Hello, you gorgeous piece of hotness."? Why do we only see the flaws, and the first thing we think is negative? We never think others look as bad as we do. We adore our friends and family and think they would look perfect covered in chicken poop and feathers.

The reality is that we are all unique, loving, sexy, hot, caring, funny, attractive, smart, beautiful, one-of-a-kind individuals. There is no one on earth like us! We are the fine wine or the aged bourbon that makes you smile as it slides down the throat!

Today's Action

Every time you look in the mirror, compliment yourself. Say things like, "Man, could you get any more gorgeous?" Don't let yourself fall into the trap of negative thought. You're only allowed to think about how fabulous you are. Notice what's right about your appearance instead of what's wrong, and don't avoid the mirror all day to get around this.

I'll warn you--this can become addictive, so if you're caught telling yourself how fabulous you are, look the bystander in the eye, smile and say they'd do well to remember it too!

Reflection Time:

- How did you feel looking at yourself with admiration and adoration instead of negativity?
- How difficult was this to do and why do you think it was/wasn't?

Throw In An 'I Love You'

What if something happened to someone you really care about and you never got to see them again? Or what if something happened to you? Wouldn't you want those closest to you to know how you really felt?

Every day is an unknown. Things happen in the blink of an eye, and your world can change. Because of this, no one in my family ends a conversation without telling the other person they love them. We also do this with our closest friends. We want everyone to understand what they mean to us.

Today's Action:

Tell everyone you care about most that you love them. They may think it's strange, so reassure them that you didn't just find out you have a brain tumor and you're dying in two weeks. If you say it regularly, they will feel comfortable reciprocating. Before you know it, the trend will spread and everyone will be saying it.

We shouldn't wait to say "I love you" until something life altering comes along. It should be an everyday conversational occurrence. I've heard arguments that you can overuse it. I laugh at the notion that you can tell someone you love them too much.

Reflection Time:

- How did it first feel when you began telling people you love them?
- How did you feel after you told them?

Personal Joy

I've never been one to pamper myself. With so many family members to think about, I'm usually at the bottom of my list. I'm also a low-maintenance, down-to-earth kind of person. I don't enjoy shopping for clothes or shoes or wear a lot of makeup. I try to live a relatively minimalist lifestyle and, overall, don't really contribute to my gender's stereotypes.

There are a few things, however, I truly enjoy and do only for my satisfaction. I keep my nails fixed and painted with my signature color, "Lincoln Park After Dark," I see my hairdresser every eight weeks, and I occasionally treat myself to a pedicure. These few things give me joy and a little peaceful me-time.

I ignored the concept that if you didn't take care of yourself, you wouldn't be able to take care of anyone else. It was only when I became run down that I began to understand how true this saying is.

You don't have to get your hair or nails done. Do whatever makes you feel happy and refreshed. Take an hour and hang out at the local book store or coffee shop. Window shop at the mall or treat yourself to a massage. Go hiking in the woods or go all out and take a pleasure cruise. It doesn't matter if anyone notices or likes it. It's a present to you from you.

Today's Action:

Do something you want to do and make sure it's only for you. Avoid feeling selfish and throw out the notion you should be doing other things for other people. No guilt allowed! Relax, be happy and enjoy.

Reflection Time:

- How did it feel to put yourself first for a change?
- What are some other things you can do for yourself?
- What are some things you'd like to try?

Truce with Time

My husband used to joke that I'd be late to my own funeral. I had every excuse in the world as to why I never showed up on time. My friends even called it *Goforth Time*.

I tried setting my clocks forward. I tried alarms. I tried every trick in the book, but time just kept kicking my ass.

Then one day, I decided to just call a truce with time and waved the white flag. I decided to quit stressing over whether I was late. I quit grinding my teeth because I had 10 minutes to get 15 miles down the road in traffic. I just chilled out and the weirdest thing happened.

First, the twitch in my eye went away and then, remarkably, I began showing up on time for meetings and appointments. It didn't happen all at once, but I slowly became friends with time. I would start my day on time and the rest of the day would fall into sync. I gave myself extra time to get to appointments and didn't schedule things so close together. I allowed time to work *with* me instead of always treating it like we were in an MMA match.

Now, I'm almost always early and *I'm* the one hearing the excuses. I always carry a book to read if I arrive with time to spare and don't freak out on those occasions when something happens and I am a bit late.

<u>Today's Action:</u>

Call a truce with time today. Look at your schedule and give yourself permission to schedule ample time between appointments to arrive early. Relax if you hit traffic. Breathe and enjoy the day. Your nerves and teeth will thank you. Also, enjoy the extra pockets of time you find from arriving early. Catch up on e-mails, read a few pages of a book, or even create a list of quick things you need to do that only take a few minutes.

<u>Reflection Time:</u>

- How was your relationship with time before this action?
- What did it feel like to call a truce with time and not be rushing all day?
- How can you incorporate this into your future schedule?

Your Mood

Do you remember when Cinderella wakes up in her little room, the sun is shining, the birds are singing and she's dancing around singing with them as they help her get dressed? Raise your hand if you want to throw up.

I'm lucky to get up and stagger to the bathroom without running into a piece of furniture and hurting myself. The only lyrics coming out of my mouth are a steady stream of grumbles with an occasional grunt unless there is pain involved and then it gets *really* colorful. So, you can imagine what my mood is like if I look out the window and see a dreary or rainy morning.

Now, I can't help if you're not a morning person (in fact, if you're not a morning person, you're my kind of people). But why do we let the weather affect our day before it even begins? We need to wake up every morning and decide what mood we're going to be in rather than letting things or circumstances dictate it for us.

Today's Action:

No matter what it's doing outside, decide to be in a good mood and have a good day right from the start. Take control of your attitude. You don't have to start your day off like Cinderella, but do what you need to do to get close to that. You can't control what happens outside, but you can control how you react to it.

Reflection Time:

- Describe the day you decided what your mood would be like. How did it feel to be the one in control instead of outside forces dictating how you felt?
- How did it feel to actually make a conscious decision of how you were going to start your day?

Possibles List

Imagine you're in a room with ten people. Each person is an expert in a different field and has ideas and thoughts they vehemently want to present to an investor. There's no order for these presentations, and each is trying to talk at once. Now, imagine you're the investor and you're trying to listen to one person while nine others are trying to get your attention. They're waving their hands and flashing shiny objects hoping you'll notice them next.

Welcome to the ADD mind! For most, it's not as chaotic as the above description, but it can sometimes feel like our minds are overflowing with thoughts and we have too much going on up there.

It's been proven that a person can only hold three to four thoughts at any given time. It feels like there is so much happening up because our mind is playing a shell game. It's moving old thoughts out and replacing them with new ones at an incredibly fast pace. In the end, however, it's still just three to four thoughts. Depending on how many items you're trying to keep track of, this constant movement in and out can create the feeling of being overwhelmed.

Because I have a lot to track, my mind is constantly shuffling through thoughts, and I have the attention span of a goldfish thanks to my ADD. So I started a possibles list. A possibles list is an ever-changing and evolving list of everything I want or need to do. It's a honey-do list for myself.

Examples of things on my list are: clean out shed (might get done), learn to change a tire (no, I don't know how to actually do this), build a treehouse for kids (I mean the 20-30 year olds), try Uncle Ronnie's compound bow to see if I want to buy one (been watching too much of The Walking Dead), get gravel for dog pen (because I'm sick of leaves in the house), replace stove in basement (for a backup heating source) and stain the house (hasn't been done in 20 years, but I'm always hopeful).

The important thing to remember is it's a *living list*. If there's something I want to do, I write it down. Once it's completed, I scratch it off. Yes, some things have taken up residence and don't seem to be going anywhere, but at least they get reviewed and not forgotten. The idea is to move the thoughts from my mind to paper so I don't have as much up there to switch around. There is also comfort that I won't forget anything because I have it written down.

Today's Action:

Start your list. Write down all the projects and things you would like to do, need to have done, fantasize about having done or intend to do. From there you can later prioritize and turn ideas into realities.

Reflection Time:

- How did it feel to get everything out of your head and listed out?
- Is there anything you can begin to turn from dream into reality?
- How often will you add to this list or review it to turn projects into actions?

Like Yourself

"Okay, I need your back straight, lower your left shoulder, turn your head to the right and your chin up. Now turn just a little more to the right and we'll compensate for your right eye being smaller than your left eye."

What? I never noticed that! Now I have something *else* to worry about on top of my butt's too big, I'm starting to get crow's feet, and my once-perky boobs are starting to want to hang with their new friend, Mr. Belly Button. I know my photographer friend didn't mean to make me more self-conscious, but that one comment is now embedded into my psyche so deep I don't know if I'll ever get it out.

Why, when we look at ourselves, does every imperfection come rushing to the forefront of our brains? The fact that you have a beautiful singing voice means nothing when all you can see is that extra 50 pounds you need to lose.

We all have imperfections. If you took a *really* good look at the prettiest person you know, you'd find their ears aren't even, they have one nostril larger than the other or they're sporting a great pair of kankles.

What would happen if we took a day and embraced everything about us without judgment?

Today's Action:

Today, love everything about you - the good, the bad, and the perceived ugly! Find a celebrity who has a similar feature than your "perceived flaw" and remind yourself of everything they've accomplished. For example, if you hate the gap between your teeth, look at Lauren Hutton, Madonna or Anna Paquin. They certainly didn't let something like that stop them from feeling fabulous.

All I have to do is look at Niki Manaj and I already feel a lot better about my rear end.

Reflective Time:

- How did it feel, for one day, to look at everything about you as a positive not a negative?
- What positives did you notice?

Happy Weirdo

My son is embarrassed at times because he says I smile and laugh too much. Are you kidding me? My reply is, "Would you rather have a mom who laughs all the time or one who's cranky?"

Life is funny. We're all funny. I laugh at myself more than anyone else. It's not that I'm an overly happy person; I just decided years ago that I would stop being a wallflower and begin looking at life a little less seriously. I began interacting with those around me to find the positives in life.

Often, we go through the motions of our day barely speaking to anyone, let alone looking someone in the eye, giving them a friendly smile or sharing a laugh. Why not?

When you notice someone smiling don't you tend to smile back? Of course-it's infectious! Why does it have to be someone else initiating that first smile?

Today's Action:

Make a game out of seeing how many people you can get to smile back at you. FYI: the Wal-Mart automotive section seems to be the toughest crowd. Be the happy weirdo. You might just be the bright spot in someone's day. How horrible would that be? Oh, and don't forget to laugh at yourself a bit, too.

Reflection Time:

- What was it like to be the one who made others smile?
- If you felt awkward, why?

Deeper Gratitude

It's easy to point out what's wrong with our lives. It's also easy to say we're grateful for blessings or gifts but I'm talking about a deeper gratitude.

Here are some things to ponder:

* Did you wake up this morning? (Check)
* Do you have a family around you that accepts you for you?
* Do you have the ability to eat each day?
* Can you smile and laugh?
* Your health may not be perfect, but are you better off than others?
* Is there someone, right now, having a worse day than you? (Like the person in the ambulance that just passed.)

* Do you make the decision of how your day is spent versus needing to spend the day meeting basic needs like food and water?
* Do you live in fear that people will storm into your house and kill you without a moment's notice like those in war-torn countries?

We can say we're grateful for the designer purse we carry around, but are you grateful for the legs that walked you to the store?

Today's Action:

Move beyond the items you listed in the action titled *Grateful List* and write down the deeper things you're grateful for. Often it's looking at this deeper gratitude that you find a real way to change your attitude about life.

<u>Refection Time</u>:

- What insights came to you as you did this through the day?
- How do you think you could continue to do this on an ongoing basis?

Long Time No See

We all have friends or relatives we would like to stay in touch with, but, alas, life always seems to get in the way. We work during the day and at night there are ball games, dance lessons, making sure everyone is fed and trying to squeeze in the last few edits of the proposal you have to give to the boss tomorrow. Before you know it, weeks have passed and your best friend is calling to see if you still remember him/her.

We can't all be like my perfectly put-together cousin who bakes cupcakes for the women's club bake sale, has time to create the perfect front door wreath and checks in with my mom more than I do, making me look like a drop-out from the Martha Stewart School of Crafts and Etiquette. I don't have a life so organized that my day planner reminds me it's been two weeks since I reached out to see how everyone in the family is doing.

Today's Action:

Call one person you haven't reached out to in a while and see how they're doing. Keep at it until you actually reach them. Leaving a voicemail does not let you check off the done box for this action! Spend two to ten minutes to chat and catch up. Let them know you were thinking about them. I promise you won't keel over from over effort and there actually *is* time in the day.

Maybe I'll call my cousin. She can tell me about the new perfectly color coordinated drapes she just bought and I'll tell her about last night's four-course meal at Steak-n-Shake.

Reflection Time:

- How did it feel to reach out to the person you called?
- How could you incorporate in your schedule to do this more frequently?
- Why do you think it took so long for you to reach out to this person in the first place?

Vision Board

Remember back in kindergarten when the teacher told the class to raid your parent's magazine stash and bring in as many as you could for the next day's school project? I always got so excited because I knew I would be cutting and gluing with wild abandon. Life was always good with glue and scissors.

We're going to revisit those days!

Today's Action:

You're going to need a piece of poster board, or a large sheet of paper. If you don't like the large paper idea, just commandeer a couple of pages in your daily planner.

Gather glue, markers, scissors (you can even use the pointy kind) and a bunch of magazines you lifted from your grandmother or mother-in-law. If you can't find any magazines because no one in your family has fallen victim to an elementary school funds drive, print off pictures. You're looking for images that represent short or long term goals you want to achieve or things you want to have.

For example, you might find a picture of the car you want to buy - cut it out and glue it on. A pile of money can mean the wealth you want to ultimately achieve. The guy with the six-pack abs can either represent the way you want to look or the guy you want to attract. You can add hearts for a great love life or things that remind you of happiness. It's your board - you decide what goes on it. There are no points for neatness, so have fun and dream big!

When you finish, you have a visual goal stimulation board, or Vision Board.

Now what do you do with it? Put it in a place you will see it daily, like on your mirror or by your bedroom door. This powerful tool is a visual reminder to keep you focused on what you want to achieve.

Note: I don't recommend doing a digital board on a computer. You lose the impact of creating the board and you can't put it above your sink to look at while brushing your teeth. You also don't get the joy of scraping glue off your fingers when you're done.

Reflection Time:

- How did you feel making the board?
- How did you feel once you finished it?
- How do you think you will feel when you look at it each day?

No Worries

We all worry. Our mother's worry about us. We worry about our children. I believe it's ingrained in us at birth. It seems the only person who doesn't worry is crazy Aunt Ester with her twenty indoor cats. She's probably the happiest person alive, but no one can stand to spend any time with her to find out.

For some of us, however, worrying has become number two next to breathing, which any doctor will tell you is absolutely horrible for your long term health. What would happen if you took the entire day and consciously didn't worry? Is it even possible? The problems will still be there tomorrow. What if you took a break? How could you even accomplish it?

Here are some ideas.

- Tell yourself you're taking a break from worrying and put it on a shelf in your brain to think about tomorrow.
- Think about other things you've been neglecting while you've been worrying and re-focus on them.
- Immerse yourself deeply in something like a hobby or movie so you don't have the opportunity to worry.
- Practice deep breathing exercises all day to relax your body and focus your mind on your breath.
- Take a yoga class. Most classes range from $2 to $10 and can be found by Googling “yoga class in [your city].”
- Wear a rubber band on your wrist and every time you catch yourself worrying, snap it to snap yourself out of it. When people stare because you’re hurting yourself all day long, just ignore them.

Today's Action:

Find a way to shelf your worries. You're on a 24-hour worry sabbatical. See what happens when you push it to the side and focus on productive things.

Reflection Time:

- How much relief did you get from shelving your worries for one day?
- What insights did you glean from this action?

Let It Go

The problem stuck in your head at bedtime that you're still thinking about this morning. The inconsiderate neighbor who can't keep their dog from taking a crap on your porch. The co-worker in the cubicle next to you who talks on their cell phone all day about things you *really* wish they didn't. It's the one thing or the one person annoying the hell out of you worse than that tickle at the back of your throat that no amount of coughing can scratch. It's driving you nuts!

As the ever-popular Queen Elsa sings in Frozen, let it go! Relieve your brain and body from this tension. It really isn't worth it. I refer to this as moving to my happy place. You just declare your independence from the annoyance and deem it will not affect you any longer. For me, I find this particularly easy to do after a Dairy Queen Heath Bar Blizzard.

Today's Action:

Think of one annoyance in your life and make the declaration that you are going to let it go. This will bother you no longer. It's all state of mind and if you deem it so it shall be. Catch yourself falling into old thoughts? Remind yourself that you're done with it and move on.

My niece has mastered this better than anyone I've ever met. She'll get annoyed and literally say out loud "Whatever, I'm over it." She then moves on to whatever she needs to do next. It's amazing how this fifteen-year-old can be so wise in the ways of stress management.

Reflection Time:

- How did you feel after just letting it go?
- How many times did you have to remind yourself that you were over it?

Negative Thoughts

This will never work! I can't believe I did something so stupid! I can't do that! I'm never going to find someone right for me! I look awful in this outfit! I'm too fat! I'm going to be stuck in this job forever! I'm never going to find what I really want to do! I'm never going to be out of debt!

Any of this sound familiar?

We walk around all day thinking negative thoughts, yet we don't catch ourselves doing it. We constantly feed on negativity - even when we're in a really good mood. It doesn't take much to derail us into AllIwanttodoisbitchville.

What if we thought things like: I'm going to make sure this works! Yea, that was stupid but I learned a really good lesson from it! I can do this! I haven't found the right person for me but I know they're out there and all I need is myself right now! I need to lead a healthier lifestyle and my reward will be a new wardrobe! I may not be happy in this job, but I will use it as a stepping stone to the one I really want! I need to spend wiser, maybe take a few classes on debt management and work on getting out of debt!

Today's Action:

On the left side of a piece of paper, write down the negative thoughts inside your head. On the right side of the paper turn the negative thoughts into positive ones you can use today. Keep the paper with you, because you're only allowed to use these positive thoughts today.

Reflection Time:

- How many negative thoughts did you catch yourself thinking?
- How did it feel to think positive through the day and throw out the negative?

Thanks

When we would eat at my Grandmother's house, I would always say Grace at the table before we dove into the food like a pack of rabid hyenas. My mom and dad weren't overly religious, but my Grandmother was another story. I would physically see her cringe when my Father threw in his end line of "Father, Son, Holy Ghost, whoever gets there first, gets the most!" Despite my father's efforts to thwart Grandma's teachings, this mealtime ritual taught me the value of giving thanks--and not just before you stuff your face.

How about thanks for the sunny day and a cool breeze? Thanks for the laugh you got when the kid with the ice cream cone ran into the door because he wasn't paying attention. Thanks for the smile from the checkout clerk instead of the usual scowl. Thanks for the phone call from a friend.

Today's Action:

We have so many little things to be thankful for and we should let the universe know. Today, say a quick thank you for all the little things that happen. It can be for something as simple as being able to reach your toes and tie your shoes after last night's ice cream fest. It doesn't matter what you're thankful for, just be aware enough to recognize them as gifts.

Reflection Time:

- What did you find in your day to give thanks to?
- What things happened to bring thankfulness?
- How difficult was it to recognize things to give thanks about?

No News

I read an article detailing a research study on how people who didn't watch the news were actually happier. I remember thinking this was probably true and, since I was pretty stressed at the time, decided to give it a shot.

That was about seven years ago and I still don't watch the news.

Am I happier for it? I have to say yes. I can boldly state this because on the rare occasions I catch part of the news, I leave feeling negative. (Sort of like kicking caffeine and then wondering why your heart is beating out of your chest from the Coke you just drank.) You have to remember that news channels aren't in business to educate you, contrary to popular belief. They are in it for the ratings! It's all about who killed whom, who died in the horrific car crash, what store was robbed at gunpoint, what child was abducted or whatever drama they can find to draw in your attention and get you to turn the dial to their station.

I'm not stupid. I know how bad things can be. Do I need daily reminders of it? No! When I walk into the office and someone asks me if I saw where a shooting occurred, I'm actually glad to say I know nothing about it.

Just so you don't think I'm completely out of touch, I do keep up with current events and I do know what's happening in the world. The difference is that I choose what to focus on by reading newspapers and a couple of online sites. I can skip completely over the negative stories or get enough details to satisfy my understanding. My weather (the great excuse my grandparents gave me for watching the news) comes from the Weather Channel app on my phone.

Today’s Action:

Give up the news. I understand that for some, this will be exceptionally hard. Turn on the music channel when you wake up instead of your politically-altered station of choice. The world will still turn without you knowing the latest tragedies, I promise. Turn off the news alerts flashing on your phone. Play music in your office instead of Before The Bell or The Today Show. We think that by being plugged in, we are connecting to the world. Un plug to see how truly connected to the world you become.

Reflection Time:

- How hard was it to unplug?
- Once you committed to it, and weren't thinking about what you were missing every two minutes, how did it feel?
- What were you able to focus on instead?

Organize

It's there, every day, waiting for you to notice and laughing at you from across the room. It mocks your goal of a completely organized life. It's the *Pile*!

Everyone has one. Most of us have three or four or 23 and counting. It's that bedroom corner by the window or the cubby next to your desk you tend to ignore and pretend isn't there. It's the shelf so packed that a speck of dust would cause it to collapse. It's the room you make sure to close tightly when company comes over.

Subconsciously, this can be a cancer eating away at your serenity. You feel frustrated knowing it's there, but it feels like organizing it would take centuries and way more energy than you have available. Besides, where would you put it?

Having clutter in our life can physically and mentally affect you. There's a sense of release and a natural high from putting things in order. Think about how good you feel when you successfully complete a project or how nice it is to be able to need something - like a flashlight - and go right to it, which, if you have teenagers, is an almost non-existent occurrence.

Today's Action:

Pick one pile, one shelf, one corner of the room and spend 10-30 minutes organizing it. Don't just take the crap and move it to another corner. Actually go through it and either keep and put it where it goes, throw it away or donate. If you're anything like me, you'll find items you've been missing for years and forgot you even had them.

This isn't about organizing everything in your life because, if you're like me, there isn't enough Xanax for that project right now. This is taking one small step. Then, if you feel better, take another little step on another day, then another and another as needed. You can take larger piles and divide them into smaller piles to tackle in increments until one day you have a space any Feng Shui decorator would be proud of. Oh, and the underlying, secondary rule here is to not create new piles to replace the old. Just thought I would throw that in there.

Reflection Time:

- How did it feel starting the project compared to how it felt finishing the project?
- How much did you accomplish? % or height?
- What other areas do you need to tackle and what will be next?

Tackle Technology

I consider myself technologically savvy, but lately I'm finding so many new programs and social media outlets that I'm starting to understand why my mother calls my son to come and fix the remote control to her television because it's too complicated.

All I have to do is spend fifteen minutes with any of my nieces or nephews to become completely flustered on what the newest craze is. How can any sane person keep up? First there is Facebook, twitter and LinkedIn. Now, I'm told these are for old people, such as me, and Instagram and Snapchat are the latest craze. I'm sure that will last for about two days before something bigger and better replaces them, if something hasn't already.

So what's the point of trying to keep up? There are two reasons other than the small part of me that refuses to give into the fact that I'm not as up to date these young whipper snappers. The first is to stay connected with what the kids in my family are into. It's the same reason I let them decide what radio station to play whenever they're in my car. I *want* to know what they are listening to. I also *want* to know how they are communicating. The world is a scary place and losing sight of what they are into can be a dangerous decision. The second is the mental benefits of learning new things. Keeping your mind active and engaged can help ward off diseases like Alzheimer's, so you're accomplishing two major benefits with one action.

<u>Today's Action:</u>

Pick a social media outlet you don't know and learn about it. All you have to do is put the title in Google and you'll be directed to hundreds of sights and videos that will teach you. Set up your own account and play with it. I did this with Instagram. I set up an Instagram account for Taz, my puppy. You can go to Instagram, look for Cutietazman and follow his crazy antics. Taz is conveniently also following my nieces and nephews so he can keep up with what they are posting--dual purpose.

Reflection Time:

- What did you learn about the program you picked that surprised you?
- How did you feel diving into something with no knowledge of how to work the system?
- How did you feel after you successfully set up your account and was using it?

Something Nice

My grandmother was very poor and lived on only $800 in Social Security each month. Before my grandfather passed in 1989, he took a mortgage out on the house, at a ridiculous interest rate, for home improvements. That left Grandmother paying a $400 monthly mortgage payment in her 80's & 90's.

Working in the nursery at church, she earned a little extra money and would babysit for neighbors occasionally. Through it all, she never complained about being unable to make ends meet.

Every once in awhile, help would come from anonymous sources. She would tell me this was God at work in her life. Sometimes it was money, but often it was food left on the porch, coming home from church to find her yard mowed or having a handy man show up to fix the busted siding on the house. Each time this would happen, she would just beam in appreciation.

My grandmother was blessed with people who loved and cared about her wellbeing. Not every elderly person we know or see is as lucky. Our society tends to avoid the elderly instead of embracing them as other cultures do.

Today's Action:

Do something nice for someone advanced in age (my grandmother hated the word elderly). It can be as simple as leaving a bundle of flowers you picked up at the grocery store on their porch or paying for the local yard boy to mow their yard so they don't have to. Everyone wants to feel cared for no matter their age. It's also wonderful to do kind acts with no expectation of acknowledgement. Brighten someone's day just because you can.

Reflection Time:

- Describe what you did.
- How did it feel to do something wonderful for someone anonymously?
- What other things could you do for someone?

No Comparing

I would *love* to look like Jennifer Lopez, but I don't see how I can succeed when I'm not Latino, I'm two inches shorter and fifty pounds heavier. I've asked my hairdresser to style my hair like hers but, as her coffee cup states, she's a beautician, not a magician. Why do I have this urge to compare myself to Jennifer Lopez and want to be like her instead of being the best me I can be?

Unfortunately, this issue starts at birth and is passed down from our parents who got it from their parents and so on. Everyone who looked at you as a baby proclaimed how cute you were, even if you had a cone shaped head, avidly declared who you looked like and the comparisons began. Mom dressed you in clothes advertised to make you the cutest kid on the block and before you knew it, you were being brainwashed. Elementary school, where most kids will play with anyone just because they're there, wasn't even safe. Parents consciously or unconsciously began to guide you toward who you should and shouldn't associate with based on their comparisons of the parents. (Don't even get me started on Toddlers & Tiaras.) When you hit puberty, with its raging hormones, and the pressures of middle school and high school, you didn't stand a chance

Today's Actions:

It's time to break the cycle! Quit comparing yourself to the guy wearing the Armani suit in GQ magazine. No matter what you do, it's impossible to look like him - and that's a good thing. Can you still be healthy? Yes. Can you still be sexy? Yes. Can you still laugh, love and have people want to be around you? Absolutely! You're no better or worse than anyone else because there is no comparison to you. It's a huge game of apples to oranges only everyone is a completely different fruit.

Focus on this today. Let it sink in. Instead of trying to be like someone else, decide what clothes YOU like to wear. How do YOU like your hair? Who do YOU want to hang out with? Be selfish for a day and really discover who YOU are. I bet you'll learn something about yourself along the way.

Reflection Time:

- Who do you compare yourself to and why?
- What did you learn about yourself during the day?
- When, specifically, did you realize you were comparing yourself to others?

Quote That Suits

"Without faith you'll give up when the going gets tough." Or "There is always time each day to progress towards your dreams." Or "There is no try. Only do or not do!" (For you fellow Star Wars geeks out there.)

We hear them all the time. "it doesn't take courage to take one step" ...yada, yada, yada. Just go to any motivational seminar, sideline of a soccer field or the staff meeting your boss is holding next Tuesday. Quotes are being tossed out like candy at a St. Patrick's day parade.

Why is this? Do they feel that by saying something inspirational, I'll see the light, raise from my seat and shout, Hallelujah, praise compliance! Why torture us with these cheesy words of wisdom?

Because, used the right way, quotes can actually be extremely helpful and motivational. The trick is, they have to mean something to you to be effective. You also have to see them more than the one seminar your sister-in-law dragged you to at the local Holiday Inn.

Today's Action:

Take a few minutes and look online, or pull from a favorite book or movie, for a quote that really resonates with you. Write, type or print it out and put it somewhere you will see every morning. Have it be something that inspires you toward a goal. My two are:

- "Think and act the way the person you want to become thinks and acts" - don't know author
- "Aut Viam inveniam Aut Facium!" - Hannibal (I shall either find a way or make one!)

These have become my mantras and definitions of how I try to live my life. That's the power of what a quote can really do.

Reflection Time:

- How difficult was it to find a quote that resonated with you?
- Where are you going to display it so you see it every day?
- How do you think you'll feel looking at it every day?

How Was Your Day?

I've tried journaling over the years, but it always seemed hokey to me. You put down your deepest thoughts at risk of having someone come along later, read them, and the next thing you know, you're having to explain why you sometimes have the urge to hold up a Hostess Twinkie delivery truck.

It's the idea of exposing yourself through writing. Putting down your dreams and desires on paper is a very personal act. I'm not ashamed of who I am, I just feel it would be better if the world didn't know *every* conversation that goes on in my head--especially after reading a steamy romance novel.

It is, however, very therapeutic to write down what you think and feel. It can release stress and relieve tension. It can also help you process issues or solve problems when you lay everything out on paper and look at situations in new ways.

Today's Action:

Write down how you felt about your day. You don't have to go buy a new journal just to try this out, a simple piece of paper will do fine at first. You don't have to write a 40-page dissertation; merely write a few simple sentences discussing what you did and how you perceived your day. It also doesn't matter if your writing technique is comparable to your second grader's. If you're overly self-conscious, you can use pictures with stick figures.

If this becomes a positive experience, maybe you'll do it again tomorrow and the next day. Before long, you'll be scouting the stores for that perfect journal and deciding if you want the leather one with the skulls or the shiny one with the Japanese flowers.

Reflection Time:

- How did you feel about the process of writing about your day?
- If not in a journal, is there some other way you can incorporate getting your thoughts and feelings out through writing?

Not Today

You know who they are. They enter the room and immediately, your left eye starts twitching. It's the one person who can ruin your day with their mere presence. The simple thought of having to deal with them makes your stomach churn like the burrito you ate the other night at the seedy, strip mall Mexican restaurant. You can't avoid them for one reason or another. They are your neighbor, co-worker, significant other of a friend or, quite possibly, related to you.

Why do we let these people have such power over us?

That's the core issue. We *let* them have control over us. We are responsible for how our body feels when we are around them. Unless they are whaling on you every time you see them, they aren't physically doing anything except walking into a room. You're doing it all to yourself.

Now, that doesn't mean they aren't the most obnoxious person you've ever met, and you would rather eat glass than talk to them. It means you are responsible for the anxiousness you feel around them and if you are responsible for it, you can turn it off.

<u>Today's Action:</u>

When you see this person, tell yourself you aren't going to let them get to you. You're going to ignore the little voice in your head that starts babbling, "Maybe if you started drinking, things would be better." You decide your mood; you decide what affects it and what doesn't. You're in a great mood and you're going to *stay* in a great mood no matter *what*.

It's amazing what happens when you take this power back. Their significance in your life tends to greatly diminish.

Reflection Time:

- How did it feel to take back your power and not let them affect the way you feel?
- How did the other person react to your different way of dealing with them?

Breakfast

Every once in, awhile I do something completely out of character. I remove the auto pilot, slow down, and have breakfast with my spouse, kids, guests or all by myself.

Whenever I suggest doing this to others, the first thing I hear is "I don't have enough time." Get up earlier! You don't have to cook a full breakfast unless you want to. A simple toaster waffle and some syrup will do the trick, or you can stop off at your local awful waffle and get it served to you. Just remember, it's not a race to see who gets done first. It's a special time starting off the day with those who mean most to you. It's taking 15 - 20 minutes out of your morning to give an extra hug and wish all a great start to a great day.

Today's Action:

Eat breakfast today and slow down to enjoy it. It's nice to pull yourself out of autopilot and experience a different way to start the day. If you traditionally eat breakfast, mix it up a bit with a new recipe or new eating companions.

Reflection Time:

- How did starting the day off slower and together enhance everyone's day?
- What did it feel like to move out of routine and slow down for the morning?

Give It Away

My husband and I are obsessed with this show called Tiny House Nation. When we're scrolling through the channel guide and see it next to Naked and Afraid, we're helpless and compelled to watch. We’re fascinated at the idea of living in a smaller footprint and giving up a large majority of the shit we’ve collected in our twenty-four years together.

Personally, I’m glad to see a growing trend of older and younger adults living with less. I look around my house and wonder, "Do I really need that eighth canister on my counter or the figurine of the bear digging into the honey pot?” The idea of having a simpler life with only what I need fills me with a joy I can't even begin to explain.

Maybe it's age or possibly the idea of never needing to go through the torture of a yard sale. Heaven!

Now, I'm far from being able to move into a tiny house right now, but I have started the process of looking at what I have versus what I actually need. I've even added a recurring to do in my book that says "What can I give away this week?" Through this process, it's getting easier and easier to find things I don't use or enjoy and give them to someone who either needs it or can love it more than me.

Today's Action:

Find one thing and give it away to someone who can use it. You can find an individual or donate it to Goodwill or The Salvation Army. It doesn't matter who gets it - just as long as you give it away. I get two great feelings from doing this. The first is the wonderful feeling that it's going to someone who needs it instead of sitting on my shelf and gathering dust; the second is the joy of not having to mess with it anymore.

I'll warn you, this can be addictive. I now actively walk into my house and scan for stuff I can give away. I even put a box in my car so that when I find things, they can go straight to it, ready for delivery.

<u>Reflective Time</u>:

- How did it feel to give something to someone who can use it or enjoy it?
- Describe the feeling you received freeing up some of your stuff.

Switch Genders

There is no denying that I'm a girl.

I have my hair done every eight weeks, nails done every three, I sew, and my crocheting could make Martha Stewart weep with happiness. I also, however, drive a motorcycle, don't mind getting greasy in the garage with my husband, and can't even explain how excited I get around power tools - I'm not talking about the tiny hand-held ones, either. There is an incredible charge when you're operating a skill saw and hacking through a piece of plywood. It' so empowering -- even if my accident-prone self needs adult supervision.

By that same token, my husband is a true man's man. He's a mechanic who I swear can pull apart and put together an entire engine with a screwdriver and have no leftover parts! He rides a Harley, has a beard that rivals members of ZZ Top, and looks like a bouncer you wouldn't want to mess with at a nightclub. He is also an amazing chef in the kitchen and can create meals that would blow your mind and "make your tongue slap your brains out".

Just because one gender typically does something, doesn't mean you shouldn't try it. Open yourself up to atypical possibilities. I know men who sew (and are the best tailors), who crochet, (a lawyer, in fact, uses it for relaxation), and women who can rebuild transmissions, (my heroes). You never know what you're going to like unless you try it. That's how my son discovered broccoli wasn't Satan's preferred vegetable.

<u>Today's Action:</u>

Pick out something you consider to belong to the "other gender" and give it a try. You might discover you actually enjoy scrapbooking or finally fixing that worn out toilet valve. You don't have to let anyone know. Just open yourself to possibilities you never explored because of the gender biases you grew up with.

Reflection Time:

- How did you feel trying something you normally wouldn't do?
- If you didn't care for it what else would you be willing to try?

Talentless?

We all have talents. Even the most talentless of us have them. We just haven't sat down to figure them up.

Here are some of mine:

- I only have to hear the words to a song once and I pretty much know the lyrics for life. (Now if I could only get on a gameshow.)
- I can drive a motorcycle.
- I have a pretty good singing voice. (I've had external confirmation.)
- I'm a beast when it comes to business.
- I can fall up any steps. (My husband still hasn't figured this one out.)
- I can carry three drinks in one hand and not spill a drop. (And that's even while walking up steps!)

- I can tie a knot in a cherry stem using only my tongue. (My husband is particularly fond of this talent!)
- I can perform the Thriller dance with 1500 other zombies down Main Street in our annual Thriller Parade.

Whether they're serious or goofy, these are my talents. They make up who I am and I'm proud of them. And falling up steps has created some great stories.

Today's Action:

Sit down and write a list of your talents. We focus so much on what's wrong with us, so this is a chance to focus on what's right. Keep the list going beyond today. I discover new talents all the time and most of them don't involve me hurting myself.

Reflection Time:

- How does it feel to notice all the great things you can do instead of focusing on the things you can't?
- Which is the most outrageous?
- Which one, if any, could you possibly turn into a hobby?

3 Things

Why is it when you really need to do something on a specific day, the universe will work to thwart you at every turn? For example, today I watched my three-year-old nephew. I also needed to pick up my husband's medicine, but he left for work with the only car seat. Since I didn't write down that I needed to pick up the medicine, the task was lost moments after thinking it needed to be done.

We are so overstimulated that our brains simply turn to mush, so sitting catatonic in a rocking chair looks like an appealing idea. We create daily task lists and fill entire pages with grandiose to-do's that have no hope of ever actually getting completed that day. Then we bump them to the next and the next until we have 1049 ideas to accomplish. By *that* point it all looks so hopeless that we live in a perpetual state of defeat.

We have to manage our days to get wins and actually *feel* like we're being productive.

Today's Action:

Pick three, and only three, things you absolutely want or need to do today. Focus only on these. All the rest can either be done in addition or wait for another day. They've waited this long already. Write the three tasks down on a post-it, type them in an app or use permanent marker and write them on the back of your hand. I don't care where you put them, but it needs to go with you throughout the day and be somewhere you will consistently see it. Your sole focus is to get these three things done. There will be no sleep until these are accomplished! Come hell or high water, you will prevail over these three things! You get the idea?

<u>Reflection Time</u>:

- How did it feel checking off the three items on your list?
- What would your life look like if you were able to accomplish three important things each day?

That Awful Noise

You can tell a lot about a person by looking at their phone playlists or Pandora stations. I'm not sure what my playlist would reveal the most, but I've got everything from Marilyn Manson to Kentucky Bluegrass to Kenny G. My tastes vary depending on my moods, which are clearly all over the board.

I've also always had the attitude that I wanted to know the music my kids were listening to. This has caused me to maintain an *extremely* open mind. Have you heard some of the stuff that's out? It is auto-tuned, auto-corrected and the only instrument is the keyboard of a computer. I've found, however, nuggets of really talented artists in genres I would have never known had it not been for my kids. Now, mind you, I've had to weed through the bad to find the good, but it's been worth it.

I've also taken a stab at listening to genres I haven't liked in the past. I figure if your taste buds change every seven years or so, then maybe your music preferences can, too - and you know what? They did for me. I now appreciate Bluegrass. I love live recordings of older bands, and I've even grown to like the sappy '70's!

Today's Action:

Turn on your child's favorite station or pick a channel you would never normally listen to for 30 minutes. Hear the music with an open mind. Don't sit there and say, "I know this is going to be a waste of time. I hate this crap." Pretend you're a music agent. Do the songs have a good beat? What messages do the songs convey? You might find that you really don't like the style of music, but at least you can say you gave it a good chance. Try another genre and see what happens there. You just might get lucky and find a new favorite song. For me, it was *Earned*

It by The Weekend. I'm not sure where he got his name, but his voice has captivated me and made me a fan for life.

Reflection Time:

- What did you think of the new music?
- What other types of music can you give a try?

The Next Disaster

The power's out. Grandpa's old camping lantern is lit, filling the cold, musty basement with dim light. Sitting on an old box of encyclopedias, I listen attentively to the voice coming through the weather band radio. My family whispers to each other as we hear the wind pick up outside. Every few minutes my mother creeps up the stairs to peek out the back window at the approaching cloud wall. The warning that caused our immediate descent to safety is expected to last another thirty minutes. The voice on the radio puts our town in the path of the tornado. All we can do now is wait.

This scenario is a yearly occurrence when you live in an area prone to twisters. At any given time, my mother can tell you exactly what our current Tor:Con threat is and what the chances are of it escalating. She knows the difference between a wall cloud and a regular storm cloud, and she can pick out a bow echo on the radar better than the weatherman. I'm not quite that hyper vigilant toward the weather, but I do understand the need to be prepared should an emergency arise. Crazy shit happens, and you want to make sure you've at least have new batteries in your flashlights.

Today's Action:

Do one thing to better prepare yourself for an emergency. I don't mean you have to go all survivalist-prepper on me, but get some bottles and fill them with water, change your flashlight batteries, or buy a few extra canned goods at the store. I went to our local flea market and bought a couple of antique glass oil lamps, then purchased some lamp oil at my local grocery store. These work great when the power goes out.

It all goes back to the old Boy Scout motto of *be prepared*. There's a great line in the movie *AVP*. The main character asks another lady why she's taking a gun on the trip to the arctic ice. Her response is, "It's like a condom. I'd rather have one and not need it, than need one and not have it." Great advice!

<u>Reflection Time</u>:

- What did you do to better prepare yourself, and how did it feel to know you had taken care of that issue?
- What are the potential threats in your area you need to possibly be prepared for?

Letter

While the shift to a technological world has its benefits, there are also some definite drawbacks; communication is one of the worst. People rarely communicate anymore. They think an email, a Happy Birthday message on Facebook or a picture with a funny caption is enough to satisfy the requirement of reaching out to others. The art of picking up the phone and speaking with someone or writing a letter is quickly drifting aside.

When my Grandfather was overseas in WWII, he wrote these amazing letters to my Grandmother. He spoke about what the war was like, the things he saw and did, how he felt and how much he loved and missed her. His handwriting makes it seem as if he's still around when I read them; I can hear his voice in the words. These letters are some of my most cherished possessions, and I'm so grateful to have found them after they both passed.

How often do you get an actual handwritten letter in the mail? How often do you even get an envelope that was hand-addressed? Anymore, these are treats when they come in our mailbox, and they're usually the first things we open.

Today's Action:

Grab a piece of paper or stationery and write an actual letter to someone you love. No computers allowed! It doesn't have to be pages and pages - just a little note to let them know you were thinking about them is enough. Oh -- remember, you'll also need an envelope and this thing called a stamp in order to mail it.

<u>Reflection Time</u>:

- How did it feel to take time and actually write a letter?
- How do you think the recipient will feel when they get it?

Grow Something

Have you heard of a *black thumb of death*? The type who could kill a cactus in a matter of days? That used to be me.

While I'm not as bad as I used to be, I tend stick to succulents and hearty plants now just to be on the safe side. I like plants, but I just have a hard time slowing down enough to realize they need water and care. If they aren't in front of me all day every day, they are kind of on their own.

So why would I have a task of growing something when I can't seem to do very well at it myself? Because I recall the excitement I felt in kindergarten when our bean plants sprouted in the milk containers. There's a sense of pride in knowing you helped a plant go from seed to sprout to plant. Further, it's a choice to slow down a bit and connect with nature, even if on a smaller scale. You're also helping the planet and teaching those around you how to care for it.

Today's Action:

Grow something! Buy a seed and plant it or get a small plant from your local garden store or grocery. If the idea of dirt doesn't appeal, take an avocado seed and suspend it in a glass of water. Watch what happens. There are so many different ways to do this action - just look on YouTube or Pinterest for ideas. A Scooby Doo Chia Pet will even work in a pinch.

Reflection Time:

- What were your initial feelings about this action?
- How do you think you'll feel watching your plant grow?

Pay It Forward

When things are going well for my husband and me, we like to thank the universe by making someone else's day a little brighter. We do this by paying for the food of the person behind us in line or conspiring with our server to cover the check of someone else eating in the restaurant. They never know who we are. and that's how we like it. It makes us feel good knowing we surprised someone and maybe created a positive ripple in the butterfly effect – (the theory that a butterfly can flap its wings in Africa and we'll get rain instead of snow in North America.)

We particularly enjoy picking up the tab for persons in the military, police or firefighters. This is our way of thanking them for their service. For the risks they take on our behalf, the least we can do is spring for their sandwich.

Today's Action:

Find a way to pay it forward. Pay for the coffee of the person behind you in the drive thru or give a few cents to the person in front of you digging in their pocket for change because they are a bit short. I'm a firm believer that what you give will come back to you tenfold. It may not be in money, but it's definitely in happiness.

Reflection Time:

- How did you feel paying it forward and doing something nice for a total stranger?
- What other ways can you pay it forward and incorporate it into your life?

Good For You

Here is my Kryptonite list (things that bring my inner Super Girl to her knees).

- Key lime pie
- Cherry Pop Tarts - iced
- The Dairy Queen Rolo or Heath Bar Blizzard
- My husband's mashed potatoes
- A Carmello bar
- Croissants of any kind
- My mother's fried chicken

If you want to see a grown woman cave quicker than a teenager snatching her dad's credit card, put one of these in front of me.

It's not that I don't like to eat healthy, I just really, *really* like these. Quite often, unfortunately, I have to stop and reboot. I physically dare anyone to have one of these Kryptonite items in my presence when I need to spend the day eating the way I should.

Once I start, it's not too hard to keep going. It's the jumping *back* on the health wagon that's the bear. Staying on the health kick gets a bit easier as I go if someone is there to hold me back from shooting myself in the foot. So far, my feet have quite a few holes in them.

Two to three days a week of being good is better than seven days of being bad, right? Man, there needs to be a twelve step program for this stuff.

Today's Action:

Make today a **reboot** day. Eat healthy and focus on not falling on your sword. Then you can say you had one good day this week. Maybe it'll turn into two and then three a week, but let's not get ahead of ourselves. Let's go for one to start.

Snickers bars, strawberry pie, apple fritters, donut holes, cheap ice cream sandwiches-- oh my God, yes - cheap ice cream sandwiches!

Reflection Time:

- How hard was it to spend the day focused on eating healthy?
- How can you add additional days to the week?

Long Way Home

Since I started consciously paying more attention to the world around me, I've noticed that everyone is in such a hurry. These days, getting from point A to point B is almost a contact sport. Cars zip in and out of lanes, cutting people off in an attempt to get one car length ahead. You're driving the speed limit, or even slightly faster, yet you're passed by others as if you were operating a horse-drawn buggy.

At what time did our life become so hectic that we need to risk it just to get home from work? The notion of a leisurely Sunday drive in the country has all but gone by the wayside.

We're racing from a stressful day at work, to a stressful drive home, to the stresses of making sure dinner is done, kids are taken to soccer practice, everyone's homework is completed, and finally, making sure the report for your boss is tied up with a nice big bow. It's no wonder road rage has almost become an epidemic.

Today's Action:

First, take a few deep breaths when you get into your car after work. Then I want you to say out loud to yourself that you don't care what anyone else on the road does. It's not going to affect you in the least. Then, I want you to take the long way home and avoid warp speed. Take a detour into the country or drive by and check out that store you want to visit but haven't because it's out of the way. Don't go your regular route home. Discover a new one. Play your favorite music or something soothing. Use this time to decompress from your day and restock your resources for the evening.

As Lily Tomlin said, "For fast-acting relief, try slowing down."

<u>Reflection Time</u>:

- Did you notice a difference in your stress levels while taking the long way home?
- How did you feel when you got home after de-stressing?

Surprise Someone

When was the last time, outside of Christmas, you were genuinely surprised by either a gift, a visit from someone special, an act of kindness, a compliment or encouraging words? How did you feel when it happened? I know every time it happens to me, I feel *wonderful*. I also know that when I'm the one giving the surprise, it feels even better.

We are all busy, but it doesn't take a lot of time or effort to surprise those around you. It also doesn't take buying the Hope Diamond. As we get involved in our day, we tend to become inwardly focused and our attention drifts away from those around us. Being the giver of small surprises reminds us to appreciate those in our lives and how special they are to us. I want everyone in my life to know they were very special to me and how thankful I am to be journeying through life with them.

Today's Action:

So what could this look like? Pick up a tray of muffins while you're at the grocery store to take to your neighbor one evening for a short visit. Write a note on a post it and put it in your spouse's briefcase or your child's book bag. Pick up a fun-looking pen and have it laying on your co-worker's desk when they come into the office. Make sure the garbage is at the curb before anyone has to notice. The possibilities are endless.

Make this a habit in your life and you'll have that wonderful feeling all the time. It's not about recognition. It's about kindness.

Reflection Time:

- How did you feel being the giver of the surprise?
- What other things can you incorporate in your daily routine to make giving surprises a habit?

Self Time-Out

Raising my two boys presented an interesting challenge when it came to discipline. I tried multiple methods with each until I found the one thing that worked, and it was different with each of them. With my oldest, it was spankings. Well, spankings might be too harsh a word. All you had to do was tap his rear and, if you were listening from the other room, you would have thought he was being water-boarded.

My youngest, however, would take whatever you could dish out and then turn to laugh at you with a look that said "Is that the best you got?" His Kryptonite was the infamous time-out. All I wanted was two minutes of stillness and 45 minutes later we were still trying. It killed him to sit still and he wasn't even ADHD!

Why is it so hard for most of us--me included--to just sit and be still?

Then, while sitting still, I'm asked to shut my brain off and stop thinking. You've got be kidding me! I've got world peace to create, not to *mention* remembering if I have cream cheese in the fridge for the taco salad I need to take to this weekend's family cookout.

Once I calmed my freaked-out brain and tossed away the notion this can't be done, however, I discovered it actually could be! I'm not saying it won't feel weird at first, but it *is* possible.

Here are the steps:

1. Sit in a comfortable position (yoga pretzel not necessary)
2. Don't think. (Having trouble? Just remember what it was like when you were a teenager.)

That's it. Really!!!

So what will this do for you? It decreases your stress, can help your body repair and run more effectively, help reduce the cortisol hormone in your body (responsible for that muffin top), and lower your heart rate and blood pressure. That's just the tip of the iceberg.

Today's Action:

Sit and just breath for ten minutes. Wipe your mind clear. Focus on feeling the air come in and go out of your lungs. If a thought pops into your mind, don't get frustrated. Just push it out and re-focus. This takes practice, so if you're not immediately a natural, welcome to the club. If you work on it, though, you'll get even better than a teenager at tuning out the world.

Reflection Time:

- How did it feel to just sit still and do nothing?
- Were you able to push thoughts from your head and just be?
- How did that feel?

Communing With Nature

There is such a feeling of peace and relaxation when you step out into nature. The calm serenity that comes from being surrounded by green can be so powerful that it drives some to give up everything and move off into the woods. Why would doing something so simple have such a powerful impact?

A study by Gregory Bratman at Stanford discovered that actual brain chemistry changes in people who took a walk in the park or woods vs. next to traffic. Those who took a walk in the woods showed improvement in their mental health, dwelling on the negative aspects of their lives was reduced, and blood flow decreased in the portion of the brain known to be involved with brooding.[4]

So, do you need to take a trip deep into the mountains where no human civilization can be found for miles? No. You can gain the same benefits by going to a local park or walking down a tree-lined street with low traffic. Even in New York City, there are places where you can get back to nature even if only for a few minutes.

Today's Action:

Find a park and take a walk. Make sure there are trees, bushes and grass. Look around and soak in the surrounding calm. Don't think about what you need to do when you're finished. Be present and notice children playing on the playground or others strolling along with you. Relax and take some well-deserved breaths. You'll be doing your brain a favor.

---

[4] Bratman, Gregory et al. *Proceedings of the National Academy of Science of the United States of America*. "Nature experience reduces rumination of subgenual prefrontal cortex activation". May 28, 2015. Vol 112 no.28.

Reflection Time:

- How did you feel walking and being surrounded by nature?
- What ways do you think you might be able to incorporate more nature into your life?

The Hidden Positive

- The line is too long at the coffee shop. I can't believe the prices they charge for a cup of coffee.
- My co-workers are idiots.
- Why am I not rich and famous?
- Why does everyone expect me to do everything around here?
- Why do I always seem to be stuck in traffic?
- Oh my God. Will they ever finish this construction?
- Why is the car making that noise? I swear - if it's broken, I'm kicking the doors in.
- I can't believe tonight is soccer practice. Why did we sign up for it in the first place?
- Why are we having meatloaf AGAIN?
- Why aren't there enough hours in the day?

Would you want to hang around the person with these thoughts? We can turn into the most negative human beings on the planet, and it usually doesn't take much to flip the switch. Then, we tend to wallow in it, searching for others to join our own little pity party. It's no wonder we have bad days; we're hanging around someone we don't even like.

The good news is that negativity isn't like a cold that needs to run its course. You have the power to stop it and instantly change your way of thinking. All you have to do is start actively looking for the positives around you. There's nothing positive, you say? Well, in kindergarten that might have been your answer as you fell to the floor throwing a tantrum. Now that you're all grown up, however, that response no longer works. There are positive things around you and you can find them. You woke up this morning, so you've got one positive already.

Today's Action:

You are to only look for positives. Notice what things are going right and put your focus there. Compliment others who make these positives happen. Get rid of that person you don't want to hang with and replace them with someone who is full of hope and enthusiasm.

Reflection Time:

- How was it different focusing on all the positives around you instead of the negatives?
- How did you feel at the end of the day not paying attention to everything negative?

Little Secret

I love Yacht Rock. There, I've said it! You now know something about me no one knew before I wrote this book.

Some - probably most - of you are saying, "What's Yacht Rock?" and others, who know what that is, are cringing and wondering why I'm actually admitting to it.

Yacht Rock is best described as 70's mellow tunes. Bands like Ambrosia, Doobie Brothers & Michael McDonald, Foreigner, Christopher Cross, Sade and Billie Ocean, etc. It's mellow, smooth and was played in a lot of 70's bachelor pads. Just imagine a guy standing in his pad, the first five buttons of his paisley multi-colored shirt undone and his gold chains glimmering from the lava lamp while *This Is It* by Kenny Loggins plays over the speaker towers in the corner. Hold onto your pants, girls!!!

I don't know why I'm addicted to it. I was born in 1970, so it's not like the songs could have had a huge influence on me at 5 years old. So, why am I admitting this? Because it's hilarious! It's a quirk of mine that makes me who I am. By sharing this with you, you now know more about my wonderful, quirky personality. We shouldn't be ashamed of the things that mold us. We should embrace our differences instead of trying to be like everyone else. I'm a proud Yacht Rock lover, I'm not ashamed to admit it, and I'm not joining a 12 step program to quit, either.

<u>Today's Action:</u>

Share a quirk or something about yourself no one knows. You can pick one person or post it on Facebook for all I care. The idea is to be fearless to say who you are or what you like. You are a unique individual and there is no one else like you. Be proud of that. It can be anything.

Have fun with it and see if you can find out new things from others you didn't know about.

Reflection Time:

- What was it like to admit something about yourself to others?
- What, if anything, did you find out about those around you that you didn't know?
- How did you feel divulging the information?

Feel The Pain

I'm writing this at the same time I'm fighting a raging sinus infection. To say I feel like death warmed over is a severe understatement. My teeth feel like they are going to burst from my mouth, and my throat is screaming from being drowned in a waterfall of never-ending snot.

We've all been here. You roll over, pop another cough drop and wonder what they'll say at your eulogy. The tissue box is empty, so to get another, you now have to lumber to the kitchen in the pajamas you've worn for three days. Making it back to collapse on the bed from the exhaustion caused by the two-minute walk feels incredible.

Sometimes, it doesn't have to be an evil virus that invaded your body to make you feel this way. It can be circumstances in our lives that have us lying in bed eating Ramen noodles and watching episode after episode of Criminal Minds. Either way, it's okay.

Today's Action:

Take the day and instead of fighting the internal pain and struggle, embrace it. Give yourself permission to wallow for **one** day. Swim in it until your fingers get all pruney and the sight of Thomas Gibson from the Criminal Minds marathon makes you hurl. Use this day to get it all out of your system, or a majority of it, and know that tomorrow, it's back to the land of the living.

Now, if you'll excuse me, I'm going to go blow my nose, pop some Ibuprofen and hope my head doesn't explode like a giant zit.

Reflection Time:

- How did it feel to give yourself permission to feel the pain for one day?

- What did you do to embrace/get past it?
- What are some other ways you can handle times when you don't feel up to fighting the day.?

Stupid Tourist

One of the greatest weekends my husband and I ever had was in Gatlinburg, Tennessee two weekends before Christmas. We were having a really rough holiday season that year and decided to just get *away*. We had no reservations and no idea what we were going to do when we got down there, so on the way, we decided to be stupid tourists. If we saw something we wanted to see, we stopped to see it. No rules, no time constraints.

It was one of the most amazing and wonderful weekends we've ever had!

We stopped at a car museum and spent two hours wandering around more classic cars than I've ever seen in one place. We went through the Ripley Believe It or Not

Museum and actually *read* all the little cards of information next to the exhibits. (Anyone with kids knows this never happens). We even stopped and made plastic molds of our hands clasped together! It was one of those incredibly magic weekends.

Now, we routinely pop into stupid tourist mode, whether in our area or when we're on vacation. When you become a tourist, you see things differently and try experiences a normal adult never would. You see the world's largest ball of twine or frying pan. You check out the local artists' sculpture garden. How many things are right around the corner from you that you knew were there but never took the time to visit? You'll be amazed at what you uncover.

Today's Action:

Pop into stupid tourist mode. Pretend you're new to the area and visit a local attraction. What would a tourist check out? What looks interesting? No rules, no time constraints.

Reflection Time:

- What new things did you discover?
- How did it feel to pop into stupid tourist mode?

Repurpose

I'm not quite Mick Dodge, living off the land and reusing everything, but I've started taking a good look at what I toss out and asking, "Can I repurpose this in some way?" If I think there might be a way, I hit apps like Pinterest for ideas.

I've crocheted bread bags into outdoor rugs, turned milk jugs into seed starters for my garden, and the pallets in my garage will make a nice outdoor bar for my deck. I even made a rain barrel in the workshop I found through Bluegrass Greensource, our local water education program. I thought I was big time!

Today's Action:

While you don't have to go crazy, you can learn to reuse some things instead of just adding to the landfills. Every little bit helps. So today, find one thing you can repurpose instead of throwing out. Find some junk in your garage or even an empty sour cream container after taco night. If you're having trouble deciding what to do with it, consult Pinterest. If you don't know what Pinterest is, beware - it's totally addicting and I can't be held responsible!

Reflection Time:

- How did it feel to know that you kept one thing out if the landfill and found an alternate use for it?
- Could you be a bit more aware of what you throw away going forward?

Look 'Em In The Eyes

Looking people in the eyes when you speak to them seems like such an easy thing to do, but it's difficult for many people because there are awkward facets to this skill. If you look too long, they're going to think you're either creepy or practicing for the county fair staring contest. If you don't look long enough, you're not interested in what they have to say or your ADD is on hyper drive.

It's no wonder we avoid it like the plague! It's almost as taboo as talking to someone on an elevator instead of quietly moving to the opposite corner, staring at the advancing numbers and pretending they aren't there.

In reality, looking people in the eyes when you speak to them is a very respectful gesture. It's saying, "I acknowledge you as a person and you have my undivided attention." Think about the last time you went through the checkout line at the grocery store. Did you actually look at the cashier and acknowledge them or did you pass through, with your head purposefully pointed down while the nameless individual scanned your items?

Today's Action:

Look everyone you meet in the eye when you speak with them. This will feel *extremely* awkward at first, but ignore the voice in your head screaming to look away. After you practice a few times, it gets easier and easier. Your credibility will increase and so will the perception people have of you. All from this one simple skill.

Reflection Time:

- How did it feel doing this at the beginning of the day vs. the end of the day?
- Did you notice people acting differently towards you?

- How did you feel looking people in the eye when you talked to them?
- Was there anything in particular you noticed about them?

Get Lost

Being attention deficit means I have a hard time focusing on tasks. I constantly leave myself reminders and my phone alarm is one of my best friends.

One aspect of this condition most don't understand is our ability to hyper-focus on certain tasks. To be super focused means to get so wrapped up that time ceases to exist. I can have someone talking right next to me and hear nothing. I can spend eight hours at my sewing table only stopping when my feet need the break. It's a zone-out of epic proportions except for what I'm focusing on. Total beast mode!

There's a meditative quality to getting lost in a task. I'm relaxed and all other voices leave my head.

Today's Action:

Get lost in something. It can be a project, a book, a video game or a part of the city or state you've always wanted to go to without any route or final destination. Just get lost. Don't say "I'm going to get lost until 3:00PM, and *then* I have to go to the grocery." Take the kids to your mother's or neighbors. This requires opening up your whole day. Get lost in a bath or a steamy romance. It doesn't matter what. You'll know if you've succeeded when the clock ceases to tick.

Reflection Time:

- What did you get lost in?
- How did it feel to push everything aside and get lost in something?
- How often in your week could you plan time to just get lost in a task?

The Extra Step

Growing up, my room could have been mistaken for a CDC hazard testing facility. Nothing *ever* made it to where it belonged. I remember my mother opening the door, letting out a huge sigh and then closing it back, unwilling to take on the challenge. I get it now. Fight the battles you can actually win!

Growing up this way did instill some pretty terrible habits that carried into adulthood. I am horrible about putting things where they go. It's so much easier to just toss the keys on the counter and kick off the shoes at the door as I throw my purse to the floor. Who needs designated spots?

Unfortunately, I can never find the things I need without turning my day into an Indiana Jones treasure hunt. I tried to compensate for this by marrying the most observant human being on the planet, and he's a godsend in remembering where my stuff is, but in reality, I shouldn't expect him to have to keep up with me that closely.

Today's Action:

You don't have to be as extreme as me, and I really hope you're not, but I'd be willing to bet there are areas where you slack off on the organizational front, too. So today, decide to take extra steps. Instead of tossing your shoes under the end table, take them to the closet. Actually hang your keys on that $40 key holder you just had to have from Bed Bath & Beyond. Make the effort to put things where they go.

And, with all that free time, you can come to my house and help me find my remote.

Reflective Time:

- Be honest, did it kill you to put stuff where it actually goes?
- How did it feel to be able to go right to a spot and find what you were looking for?

Saying Grace

My father was raised Southern Baptist and my mother Catholic. Apparently neither of my parents were enamored with their upbringing, so I grew up in a household where the closest thing to saying grace at the table was my father proclaiming "Father, Son, Holy Ghost. Whoever gets there first gets the most," or " Good food, good meat, good God, let's eat!"

When I first read about the benefit of saying grace before a meal, I found it rather hard to buy into because the practice had never been a part of my life. The more I thought about it, however, the more sense it made.

Grace is meant to send positivity and gratitude into the universe. Since everything is made of energy, saying grace over your meal infuses the food that nourishes your body with positive energy. In my opinion, this can only do good things.

Today's Action:

I don't believe you need a long or flowery declaration and saying grace doesn't have to be rooted in any religion or directed at God. A simple thank you to the universe for what it's provided is sufficient. I also believe you don't have to say it out loud. You're merely slowing down, paying attention to what you're eating, who you're eating with, and giving a little thanks.

Reflection Time:

- What did it feel like to slow down, pay attention and give thanks for the food you ate today?

Stuff Around You

I can pay bills, access my bank account, and see what's showing at the movies tonight while destroying buildings with flying birds that explode - all from my phone. I can print from across the room with no wires and can have any movie I want appear on TV with the touch of a few buttons. If I can't find a movie I like, I have 900 channels to choose from or I can turn off the TV and choose music from a library of a million songs. My coffee maker can have my coffee done by the time I crawl out of bed and my new pressure cooker can cook a tender roast in an hour. We can hop on a piece of metal that will take us in the air and land across the country in a matter of hours. We're close to living in a Jetson's world.

We have so many gizmos and gadgets that make our lives easier, and we rarely take the time to appreciate them. Have you ever had to experience no indoor plumbing? Have you carried your water up from a creek? Built your own house or grown your own food? Have you seen what a lawn mower looked like before engines?

Today's Action:

Pick one piece of technology you use daily and go without it for a day. Go old school. This is a great way to maintain gratitude and sometimes the old ways are actually better than the new. This is also a great way to teach youngsters how life was before the conveniences they now have and take for granted. It will also come in handy when the zombie apocalypse hits and the grid goes down.

Reflection Time:

- What items that make your life easier are you grateful for?
- What would your life be like without them?

- What is something your grandmother or grandfather had to do that you are grateful you don't have to do today?

Get Out Of The Zone

I have a favorite quote that says, "You have to scare the crap out of yourself on a regular basis."

I like this quote because it reminds me to truly live. As I got older, I noticed I didn't take as many chances as I once did. In my 20's, I did stupid things all the time. As I began experiencing pain, hurt, fear, and regret, I shielded myself in a cocoon of what was safe and known. I had children and responsibilities. It wasn't right or proper to act irresponsibly. Slowly, however, the vitality and adrenalin rush of taking chances waned.

As you ease into this concept, I would recommend not doing anything overly-dangerous like bungee jumping or skydiving, unless that's a must do on your bucket list. I personally cannot understand why anyone would jump out of a perfectly good airplane, but I'm not here to judge. That said, you can scare the crap out of yourself in many much safer ways. Speak in public (although some would consider this far worse than skydiving). Ask the girl or guy of your dreams out for coffee. Ride a motorcycle. Or, do what I did and give up your 20-year corporate career to start your own business. Talk about scarier than skydiving.

Today's Action:

Do something out of your comfort zone. It'll be hard and you'll probably call me every name in the book, but when you're finished puking you'll truly feel alive. You went for it, despite outcome. Now, you just have to learn to do it more often.

Reflection Time:

- How did you feel before you stepped out of your comfort zone vs. after?
- What other ways could you step out of your zone?

Another Language

I *love* other languages. Communicating with friends when no one else understands the conversation just brings out the devil in me!

I'm currently trying my knack at Irish, Spanish & Russian. Spanish because it's all around me, Irish because of my heritage and I plan to visit Ireland in a few years, and Russian because I've always found it to be a beautiful language when spoken, and I'm intrigued with the challenge of learning a language from a different alphabet.

I've never understood the mentality some have that everyone should just learn English. What's wrong with being able to say "Hello" or "Goodbye" or, heaven forbid, "Please" and "Thank You" in another tongue? I'm not talking about translating at a United Nations Peace Summit, but I at least want to be able to order a beverage and ask where the bathroom is. Also, studies have shown that learning other languages is a great way to create new neural pathways in your brain, which can delay or prevent Alzheimer's.

Today's Action:

Grab your phone, pick a language you've always found interesting, download a free app, and start with simple words and phrases. It's not as hard as people make it out to be.

Just remember, это все о сохранении непредвзято! (It's all about maintaining an open mind!)

Reflection Time:

- What did it feel likely be able to say a couple of phrases in another language?

- How, or where, do you think you would be able to use them?

Something Daring

I'm at the Women Leading Kentucky conference and the motivational speaker starts talking about the need to do something daring that no one around you knows about. Something that's just your little secret. It could be as bold as getting a tattoo in a spot no one would see or as mild as wearing two different-colored socks. Hell, it could be wearing naughty, superhero or even no underwear.

Since one of my actions is to step out of my comfort zone, I chose to go commando. This admission is probably way too much for my co-workers to handle, but they never knew what day I did it so they'll eventually be alright.

What happened was amazing. The entire day I had this crazy sense of power. I knew something no one else knew. I had more energy, worked like a beast, and was more productive than I had been in a long time. It was one of the most amazing challenges I've ever tried.

<u>Today's Action</u>:

You're going to do something daring today that only you know about. Ladies, you're going to go commando. Men, you're going to pull out those boxers that have "Love Machine" written all over them. Remember, you can't tell anyone. It's your secret. Have fun with it and see what happens. If you experience anything like I did, everyone will wonder why you're in such a good mood and have that evil smile on your face.

<u>Reflection Time:</u>

- What were your first reactions when you read about this action?

- What did it feel like to go all day with a secret no one else knew about?

There Is A Plan

Growing up, hearing my mother and grandmother talk about where they were when Kennedy was shot or when the astronauts landed on the moon always seemed weird. How could something be so embedded in their memory?

I am writing this action on September 11, 2015 at 8:30AM. Fourteen years ago to the minute the first tower had been hit, people had lost their lives, and I finally know what my mother and grandmother meant. I remember exactly where I was at this time. I had just dropped my niece off at daycare and was headed into work, everything unfolding on the radio as I made my way through traffic.

I fundamentally believe everything happens for a reason, but often it's difficult to understand what that might be. As I look back at that day and the subsequent tragedies in my family, it's hard for me to grasp that horrific things can happen, let alone find meaning in them. I've learned, however, to take each tragedy and try to learn from it, no matter how small. I've learned not to take the small things for granted. I've learned to live each day as full as I can and I've learned the power of a simple phone call to say *hello* and *how was your day*?

Today's Action:

Look at the things that have happened in your life. Get out a sheet of paper and write down what lessons have you've learned from them. Then ask yourself the following questions. How are you different because of these experiences? Is there something connecting these that's pushed you to be the person you are today? Is there something more you need to be and haven't embraced? Don't just look at the bad--see the good, too.

I believe there is a purpose for each of us being here. Our job is to look in our hearts, learn from what's around us, do what we feel is right, and have faith in ourselves.

<u>Reflection Time:</u>

- How did it feel to look at things from this perspective?
- What revelations did you have?

Commit

I've lived in the same house for 23 years. I've been married to the same man for 24 years. I drive vehicles until they have 300,000 miles on them. I was at the same job for 20 years. My husband tells me I have real commitment issues.

It seems for all the really serious things in my life, I can commit like no other; ask me to finish a small project, and you're looking at a completely different woman. I currently have five afghans I'm crocheting and four books I haven't finished reading. There are about ten sewing projects I've either started or need to start and I have only one or two rooms in my house that don't have some level of renovation going. Don't even get me started on the list of things I *want* to do. I'm great at starting something, but I suck at committing to finish.

Why is it so hard to commit to things? For me, part of the problem is that I'm easily distracted. The other issue is the time commitment. Some projects just take an inordinate amount of time. By the time I'm halfway done, I'm bored with it. Thank goodness I've never gotten bored with my husband!

Today's Action:

Commit to something with every ounce of your being. Jen Sincero, author of You Are A Badass, gives the best description I've ever heard. She says go for it with the passion of "a dateless cheerleader a week before prom."[5] If it's a project, finish it. If it's a decision you need to make, make it. Go all in or go home. Find your prom date!

[5] Jen Sincero. *You Are A Badass* (Running Press, 2013). 164

Reflection Time:

- List things you have yet to commit to of finish.
- How do you feel about the list?
- How did you feel committing to one thing all in?

Learn Some History

In seventh grade, I had a history teacher who was obsessed with the Civil War. She ate, drank, breathed and bathed in it. She made us create a booklet where we charted every battle or conflict, who fought it, where it was, what the major outcomes were and who won. It was the most amazingly insane thing I've ever had to do for American History. The room was divided into the North and the South, and we had to debate between each other constantly. It took an entire semester just to study the one war.

Of course, since it was seventh grade, the one thing I really remember is when she discussed the wounded. The term "bite the bullet" came from the war because they would run out of morphine, and men literally had to bite a bullet to endure the pain of getting their arm or leg amputated. Some hospitals had limb piles two stories tall. Surgeons would simply throw the body parts out the window once they finished hacking away. We spoke about Gangrene and all the horrible diseases the men could contract. I even remember the vivid details of the foot issues the men had to endure as they marched across the land. It was stomach churning, but it was one of the best classes I ever had.

This lady had classroom after classroom enthralled with the civil war - a topic most couldn't recall even if they had a cheat sheet. Now, not every history class I took was like hers. Believe me--I've drooled through many others as I bobbed in and out of consciousness; however, as I've gotten older, I've begun to appreciate history much more. I started visiting local historical sites and discovered battles, inventions, and a world of information I never knew about right next to me.

Today's Action:

Visit somewhere historical in your area and learn about it. Make it fun. Go on a ghost tour with friends if your town has one; these are full of historical information. See if your town has a historical society or museum you can visit. You can even go to your local library and peruse the stacks. Just look up something you think might be interesting and learn a little bit about it. There is wisdom in knowing where we came from to help us know where we need to go.

Reflection Time:

- What did you pick to learn about and what facts did you find?
- How did you feel taking the time to do this action?

<u>Curious</u>

In a prior life, I must have been a cat, because my curiosity knows no bounds. Now that I think about it, that's probably why I'm no longer a cat. I think the curiosity stems from my love of learning. I have no specific topics I stick to. I can converse about all sorts of things, from website design all the way to Ancient Aliens. With me, the sky's the limit.

I recently discovered Coursera. Through Coursera, major colleges get tax breaks to offer college-level courses for free online. There are *hundreds* of courses you can take either just for fun, or, if you qualify, you can receive a certification of completion to go toward college credit. It doesn't matter what your current education level is; it's open to anyone who can get on a computer. It's amazing how the internet is changing the way we learn--knowledge is no longer held by an elite few.

Learning should never stop when school ends. You should learn something, no matter how small, every day of your life. Great leaders and the country's wealthiest individuals will tell you they never stop discovering new things. It's the cornerstone of how they became successful.

Today's Action:

Pick a subject or skill you've always wanted to learn about and discover it. I don't care if it's pygmy head-shrinking. Just take a few minutes and create new neural connections in your brain--like learning a new language, this is said to be one of the greatest defenses against Alzheimer's. It also won't kill you. Unless you're a cat.

Reflection Time:

- Why did you pick the topic you picked to learn about and what did you discover?

- What did it feel like to learn something new?
- How can you learn something new every day/week/month?

Take A Chance

Everything we do involves some type of risk. You wouldn't think getting out of bed in the morning involved risk until you trip over the dog toy on your way to the bathroom, arms flailing as you fight to stay upright. Our brains weigh these risks, either consciously or subconsciously, and alert us about potential trouble should the risk outweigh the reward.

Every once in awhile, however, you need to ignore your brain's warning and say, "to hell with the consequences, I'm going for it." Take a chance, roll the dice, stick your neck out, play with fire, run with scissors, ask for trouble, skate on thin ice, pluck up and move forward with bold enthusiasm.

Today's Action:

Today is the day to take a chance on something. Ask for the raise, invite someone you like out to dinner, accept that job you feel you have no idea how to do or go for one that you think you'd love. Be bold and remember: it's not about the outcome. Whether it works out or not, it's about you looking risk in the eye and telling it you're ready for the challenge. Be empowered to move beyond what's comfortable. Pull that inner daredevil out and let her/him run free for a bit. Ask what if? or why not? The power of bravery is immense and wonderful. If you can muster up the courage to take a chance on this, what else are you capable of?

Reflection Time:

- How did it feel to take a chance?
- How can you incorporate taking more chances in your life?

It's A Good Day

There are times when I decree that no matter what happens, my day WILL be a good one. Murphy's Law can throw it's best at me and I won't be phased one bit. I will laugh at all attempts to thwart my decree and barrel through them like The Road Warrior.

Even through my morning-fogged mind, I've done this many times. It's all about focus. The one thing you can control in any situation is your attitude. *You* decide to get mad when your day dissolves to a pile of moldy, wet leaves on a bleak, fall day. You also decide when nothing can ruin your happiness.

Today's Action:

You're going to deem today a good day. The moment something negative happens, you're going to catch the enemy thoughts creeping in and kick them to the curb. Positivity is the *only* emotion you have time for today.

This won't be easy, but it will happen. Tomorrow you can decide if you want to go back to being Murphy's victim. Today, he's the old ex you forgot all about.

Reflection Time:

- How did it feel kicking negativity to the curb for a day?
- What steps did you take?
- How can you incorporate a bit of this into every day?

Deep Thought

Whenever I hear the suggestion to think deeply, I imagine two guys sitting in their basement, smoking weed, and talking about an entire universe existing in a speck of dust under their fingernails as they munch on potato chips. It's that whole "Horton Hears a Who" concept.

When the giggling in my head subsides, however, I realize the power of taking 10-15 minutes and thinking about how amazing things really are. Take our bodies, for example. We are made up of trillions and trillions of cells. Each one operates exactly as it was designed to do in harmony with everything around it. The collective result is that we can breathe, think, see, communicate and do the lawn sprinkler dance because those cells work together in perfect harmony. When you think about it, each of us really *is* a walking miracle.

So, if we're already miracles, what else are we capable of? Looking at things from this 30,000-foot perspective minimizes everyday issues and opens possibilities. When compared to the magnitude of what your trillions of cells are already doing collectively, writing that book or learning to woodwork looks like a cakewalk.

<u>Today's Action:</u>

Sit down and take ten minutes to really think about this concept. Then, on a piece of paper, write down what you feel you're capable of doing and the issues holding you back. Then, take each issue and think about how, not if, it might be overcome. From a deep thinking perspective, you've already overcoming obstacles so great that anything you list should be a piece of cake.

Reflection Time:

- How was thinking this way different than you've thought before?
- What revelations, if any, did you have about what you would like to do?

Energy Suckers

I love vampires. I'm a HUGE Anne Rice fan, and there probably isn't a vampire movie or show I haven't seen at some point. This is one of my quirks I've come to embrace. It's been with me since childhood, and I don't seem to be ready to grow out of it any time soon.

On-screen vampires are fine, but in real life, they suck!

Do I think they are real? Absolutely! Do I think they drink blood? No. Vampires are our daily encounters who drain the life and energy from us just by being near. They are the constantly negative people that zap any motivation we had, leaving us mere shells in their wake. You know who they are. They are the ones that cause our bodies to cringe and tire at the mere thought of seeing them. After spending ten minutes in their company, we need a nap. I've dubbed these people Energy Suckers.

They can be friends, co-workers or even family. They however find fault in everything, exude negativity, and couldn't muster up a true word of encouragement if their life depended on it. I'm actually getting tired just writing about them. It's not that they don't care about you; they just suck and cannot/will not change.

I've only found two ways to deal with these people.

1. Avoid them
2. Arm yourself well to defend against them

If you can't avoid them, then defending against them is your best option. You can do this by first recognizing who the Energy Suckers are around you. Make sure your motivation and energy levels are high whenever you have to be together. Build a defensive shield around yourself and remember that their own life's walk should have no influence on yours. Also, don't feel bad if you just can't handle being around them. Give yourself permission to take care of you.

Today's Action:

List the energy suckers in your life, and next to each name, decide if you're going to avoid or defend against them.

Reflection Time:

- Who on your list of energy suckers was a surprise?
- What specific strategies can you put into place to keep your energy positive when around them?

Another Religion

The topic of religion is such a landmine that many just avoid talking about it. Everyone has a belief about what happens when we die. The problem is, until we die, we won't truly know which belief is right. Maybe everyone is. Maybe no one is.

Each of us is either born or comes into our religious beliefs differently. Many wars have been fought and many people have died declaring theirs is the only true way. I take the attitude that if everyone believes they are correct, then who actually is?

There are common threads through each religion that, I believe, could serve to pull us together instead of drag us apart. The issue is you have to *know* about the other religions to see these threads. You also have to see the other side with an open mind. See the problem?

I am in no way asking anyone to understand or condone atrocities done in the name of religion. What I am suggesting is that many misconceptions and differences could be put aside with a little education. I've overheard criticism of religions that, if the person criticizing had bothered to do a little homework, just wasn't factually true. This goes from differences between large categories like Christianity, Judaism, Islam and Hindu to differences between subcategories like Baptist, Catholics, Protestants and Pentecostals. When you don't educate yourself, how do you know what the other side does or does not truly stand for?

Today's Action:

Pick a religion or subset that isn't yours and learn a little bit about it, maintaining an open mind. See how they are different *and* similar. Remember that many people were raised with this belief just as you were raised with yours. If we can look for the ways we are similar, maybe things would get a little easier.

<u>Reflection Time</u>:

- What differences and similarities did you find to your beliefs?
- How would learning about other religions make you feel?

Nothing Negative

Can you go without thinking or saying anything negative for an entire day?

It's natural for us to think negatively at certain times. It's only when the negativity takes over and outweighs the positive that we have to stop and take a good look at ourselves.

There is an energy principle known as The Law of Attraction. This law explains that like attracts like and can be demonstrated using two magnets. The like poles will pull together while the opposite poles repel each other. *The Secret* by Rhonda Byrne was written primarily around this principle. Everything in the universe is made up of energy--including us. If we are positive, positive things will be attracted to us. Likewise, if we are negative, we will attract negative. It sounds like science fiction mumbo, but it's true. The things in our lives are a direct result of the energy we emit to the universe. If you want to change things, you have to start by changing the way you think and act.

There are times when we are naturally positive, like during the holidays, anticipating a date or standing on line at our favorite ice cream parlor. The ultimate goal would be for positivity to become the go-to emotion always -- no matter what happens.

Today's Action:

From the time you get up to the time you go to bed, there can be only positivity. No negative thoughts or actions allowed.

"This is never going to work," you say. BEEP! There's negative thought #1.

Keep a piece of paper with you, or record on your phone, every time you catch yourself turning negative. At the end of the day, you'll be able to see just how often your thoughts go dark. This will show what it's like *with* you paying attention. Imagine what it's like when you're not.

Reflection Time:

- What did it feel like going an entire day thinking and talking only positive?
- How many times did you catch yourself going negative and what revelations did you make from it?
- How did you counteract negativity?

Oppose Nothing or Decide Everything

I can be a control freak, and typically don't like things decided for me. On the D.I.S.C. psychological profile, I'm a hard core, to the bone, D:Driver. This means I make decisions very fast, and I only need the vital information to do it. Surrender is not in my vocabulary, and I naturally tend to step up to a leadership position in a group. It's not that I need to get my way all the time, I'm just a very strong-willed person.

So going a day without opposing anything, and letting others make my decisions, was particularly difficult. I recognize, however, that sometimes I need to surrender control and let other's ideas and opinions shine. It's not always up to me.

Today's Action:

If you are the type of person, like me, who steps up and is the decision maker, stop. Let someone else make all your decisions today – and I mean everything! Someone else gets to decide what you wear, eat and do. They even get control of the remote for the night. Be sure to pick someone you trust who won't make you wear that awful paisley shirt you should have thrown away back in the '80's.

Likewise, if you are the person who has most things decided for them, you get to step up and make all the decisions today. Come out from under your shell and accept the challenge. This isn't an opportunity to go power hungry, though. Remember -- "With great power, comes great responsibility." Not to mention paybacks are a bitch, you know.

Reflection Time:

- How did it feel either giving up control or taking control for the day?

- What discoveries did you make about yourself through this action?
- How can you find a happy medium going forward?

Make It Happen

One trait I proudly embrace is being a mousetrap builder. If someone says something can't be done, I'll try to make it happen. It's always been in my nature to do this. I don't accept defeat until I've exhausted every avenue of possibility.

If everyone gave up when finding solutions got difficult, we'd be in a world of hurt today. We also wouldn't have light bulbs, telephones, smartphones or swim fins if it weren't for Thomas Edison, Alexander Graham Bell, Steve Jobs and Benjamin Franklin doing what others said was impossible.

Today's Action:

Build a better mousetrap for something deemed impossible. See what happens. Maybe they're right, or maybe you'll bring a different way of thinking to make something happen. Often, problems only need a thought shift to turn impossible to possible. The word impossible is made up of I'm Possible.

Reflection Time:

- What was your mousetrap?
- Whether you were able to make it happen or not, how did it feel to take on the challenge and look at things from a new perspective?

A Reason

I don't believe everything happens for a reason just for the big events that happen in my life. I believe our days are full of happenstance. You just happen to be standing in the same line as one of your best friends from school who you haven't seen in years, or you just happen to be next to the mechanic's shop right as your car starts to make a screeching noise like it's been attached by a pack of rabid gremlins.

Many believe in guardian angels, and perhaps they are real and working to keep us safe until we fulfill our purpose. If it's true, I've definitely had mine working overtime on occasion.

Others will say it's just blind luck. At some point, usually when my frustration is at its highest, I've learned to step back, breathe, and realize my way is just not supposed to happen. At that point, I surrender and go with the flow. Once I do this, a calm comes over me and my stress levels decrease.

<u>Today's Action:</u>

Let everything unfold today as if it's meant to be. There's no sense in struggling when it's just not meant to happen. Be ok with that. Consciously say to yourself that there is a reason for what's happening. Then thank the universe or God or the angels for watching over you.

<u>Reflection Time:</u>

- How hard was it to catch yourself tensing and reign it back in to go with the flow?
- How did it feel to just accept that there is a reason you weren't meant to do something?

No Angst

Will I ever find my true career? My soul mate? My purpose? How am I going to pay my bills? Will my car make it another two years? Why is my family so crazy? When will I have my own place?

The frenzy is here. We get caught in an angst loop because we don't have the immediate answers. Our minds take over and we worry until we have to spend fifty-five dollars on a cream that promises to reduce our worry lines. Is there anything we can do at *this moment* about them? Probably not.

So why can't we let them go for a bit and allow our brains and nerves enjoy a well-deserved vacation? The questions will still be there tomorrow. They won't disappear. Sometimes, we simply need to put worry aside. Worry is the future that hasn't unfolded. We have no way of knowing whether events will occur as predicted – or, the more plausible scenario, they will be far different and a lot less dramatic.

When we spend time worrying, we are spending time in an imaginary future. We aren't paying attention to the present.

Today's Action

Put all your unanswered questions to the back of the line. They will still be there when you decide to revisit. Notice what's actually happening at *this* moment and what *you* can do *now*. The worry can return tomorrow unless today is so wonderful that you decide to extend the vacation a bit longer.

Reflection Time:

- What did it feel like to put all the burdening questions to the back of the line and focus on what was actually happening now?
- Instead of having the angst with you all day every day, is there a time when you might be able to review them and then tuck them away so you don't stay in an angst loop?

Walk In Their Shoes

There is a song I grew up with called "What It's Like" by Everlast. If you're not familiar with it, I would suggest looking it up. It's about putting yourself in someone else's shoes before judging them. It's easy to say "Well, if I were them I would/wouldn't _____." But the reality is that you can't know – you're not them.

It's too easy to judge someone based on how you feel you would react, but you are different with different experiences. Of course you probably would do things another way.

Today's Action:

Before you internally judge someone, take a few minutes and see if you can put yourself just a little bit in their shoes. The young mom with the screaming kid at the grocery store. The grumpy coworker who you don't get along with. The high school student with the four-foot Mohawk. The homeless guy on the corner. It's easy to fall into judgement. It's much harder to understand, forgive and accept.

Reflection Time:

- How were you able to put yourself in the shoes of another person?
- What did you discover about them and yourself in doing this?

Be A Kid

Think of that story when you were a kid that your mom loves to tell family members - and total strangers - around the holidays or at random opportune times throughout the year.

Mine begins with my brother and me playing too quietly outside. Now, as a parent, I understand that this immediately arouses suspicion. Upon further investigation, my mother discovered us in the middle of the mud puddle that had formed at the end of our driveway after a particularly heavy rain. Kids will always play in mud puddles, but I had taken it to a whole new level. To me, the puddle was a bakery and I had made numerous mud pies that just had to be sampled. My customer was my little brother.

The story goes that he was found lying in the puddle with me sitting on his chest shoving mud pies down his throat. He couldn't scream for lack of air due to the mouth full of mud and my method of keeping him contained. Personally, I don't remember the incident; however, I do know how stories get exaggerated over time, so I don't think he was as close to death as is told.

The important thing to remember is not that I almost killed my little brother. It was the '70's and that happened on a daily basis. Back then, we didn't even wear seatbelts! But that I was in the *moment*. I had that bakery open and I was making mud pies so good they needed to be eaten. My imagination was going wild, and it was great to be a kid. There were no deadlines, bills, appointments or responsibilities. My only worry was if I brushed my teeth before bedtime.

Today's Action:

That feeling is still in us. It may be buried pretty deep, but it's there. Today, I want you to think about what it was like when you were a kid. Really dig deep and pull out that creative and powerful energy. Then share that feeling with someone close to you. Tell them a funny story, or go out and actually *swing* on a swing set. Relive for a bit what it was like to truly live in the moment and play a little.

Reflection Time:

- How did it feel to think back to when you were in the moment all the time? How difficult was it to pull out?
- What activity can you do going forward to bring out your inner kid regularly?

Be Fearless

What would you do if you had no fear? If you went through your day with a "Why not?" attitude? If you didn't let fear keep you from your dreams?

You'd be pretty unstoppable.

So why do we let fear take control so easily? I understand self-preservation, but I'm not talking about jumping off a bridge tethered to a rubber band. I'm talking about the non-life threatening fears that control us daily. "What if they don't like me? What if my idea is shot down? What if she/he says no?"

We can't predict the future no *matter* how hard we try, but we live in this imaginary future where the worst things happen. If you acted fearless, the odds of the worst happening every time is pretty remote.

Today's Action

Be fearless. Go for things you would normally shy away from. If things don't go great, so what. You at least *tried!* Wayne Gretzky said "You miss 100% of the shots you never take!" Take those shots today.

Reflection Time:

- How did it feel not letting fear run your day?
- Describe how you were fearless.
- What can you do on an ongoing basis to keep this fearless attitude?

Future Dilemmas

The Power of Now by Ekert Tolle, proposes that we spend a lot of time either in the past, which has already happened and can't be changed, or the future, which has yet to happen and is not set in stone. All you actually have is *right now*. If you spend time in the past or future, your present is gone.

Every once in a while, you come across teachings that change your thinking and perceptions. This book deeply resonated with me because I spent a lot of time worrying about the future and what was out of my control. My inner control-freak hated this. I would think about it so much that I physically felt sick and drained. But let's be honest -- if anything actually happened, it was often so much less dramatic than what I had envisioned in my head. I was doing all this worrying for nothing.

Today's Action:

I'll warn you; for some, this won't be an easy task. Clear your mind of all talk and notice what is right in front of you. Enjoy being in this moment. Nothing is happening right now except you're reading this book. Feel the pages and its weight in your hands. Notice your breathing. Do you hear the furnace or the television in the other room? Feel the seat below you. Take each of your five senses and see what messages you are receiving through them.

Reflection Time:

- How hard was it to move the past or future from your mind?
- What senses did you get from your five senses? Touch? Taste? Sound? Sight? Hearing?
- How is this sensation different from how you regularly go through your day?

Focus

We live in a world of constant distractions. When we drive, we're bombarded with billboards and signage *everywhere*. Our phones beep and buzz and we immediately check our e-mails or texts. If there's a piece of information we can't remember, Google can provide it almost instantly. Want to know that song on the radio? Shazam it. Commercials cut into our shows, our radios, and our lives. Our world is one giant distraction, so it's no wonder we have trouble focusing on one thing at a time. I don't see how the children growing up are ever going to know any other way.

Today's Action:

Find one thing you need to accomplish. You are going to focus on it and nothing else for a period of time. If you can get it done in the amount of time you decide, wonderful. If you can just move a little further toward completion, excellent. Silence your cell phone and keep it in a drawer. Turn off the TV and radio. Cut yourself off from everything except your task. You may be antsy, but keep going. It just takes practice and it *does* get easier the more you do it. Eventually, you'll be getting more done that you ever thought imaginable, and you won't miss seeing a single ad.

Reflection Time:

- What differences did you notice in your focus when you got rid of all the distractions around you?
- What distractions do you have on a daily basis?
- How, going forward, can you limit these distractions so you focus more going forward?

Be More

We are creatures of habit and victims to routines. We get out of bed each day, get dressed, and head off to work. Some of us stay home and care for kids or loved ones.

Every once in a while, for reasons we may not understand, we can have days where we are supercharged. We feel great, we're productive, and the world is our oyster. We may laugh about how it doesn't happen often, enjoy it, and then fall back into the same routine the following day.

Why does it have to be random occurrence, and why don't we get to choose when? I believe that at any given time, we have the power in us to *be* more. To be more of the mother and caregiver. To be more at our careers. To push ourselves to do better than we did yesterday and plan to be better tomorrow. Why can't it be our decision?

Today's Action:

Be more at whatever you do. Put that little bit of extra something into every task. You'll work harder, laugh louder and love stronger. Be the best you possible. It's surprising when you see just how incredible you really are when you let your inner greatness out.

Reflection Time:

- How were you able to be more today?
- How did it feel to make the decision to be more?

Brain Dump

It has been scientifically proven that our brains can only hold three thoughts at a given time.

I'll bet you're probably doing what I did when I first heard this. I rolled my eyes in disbelief, laughed, and thought there are way more than three going on in my head. When my ADD is in high gear, it can sound like the paparazzi at a red carpet event – everyone screaming, trying to get my attention.

What I didn't realize is that while there are only three thoughts, they are constantly being replaced over and over like the cup game you see at carnivals. This constant replacing makes it feel like you have way more in there, but it also means thoughts don't stay in your head for long.

Maybe you'll come back to them or, in my case, maybe you won't.

That's why it's so important to get things out of your head and written down in a journal, day planner, or the stack of post-its currently gathering dust in the back corner of your desk drawer. Too much information can create a sense of being overwhelmed, which causes stress. It's only when you do a "brain dump" that you can sit down, calmly look at everything you wrote, and create action steps.

"But won't I get stressed when I see everything written down in front of me?", you ask. While the list, for some, may be daunting, it's minimizing the constant repetition in your head by adding the ability to create a plan around how to complete tasks, to reduce stress. You no longer have to worry about forgetting something because you've got it down. All you need to do is add as you think of things. This alone was a *huge* relief for me.

Today's Action:

Get something you can keep with you to make a list, or several if you're like me. Sit down and do a brain dump. Write down all the things you need to do this week, all the things bothering you, all the ways your brother annoys you. It doesn't matter, just get it out. If you're like me, you'll be amazed at how much you have rattling around up there.

Reflection Time:

- How did it feel to just get everything out of your head and written down so you don't have to remember it anymore?
- How are you going to prioritize it so you can complete some of the things you need to do?

No Drama

Drama! Everyone says they hate it, but it haunts our days and nights like a bad episode of Dallas or The Jersey Shore. Just look left or right the next time you're in a checkout lane. All you see is who did what to whom, who is having whose baby or who got drunk, cheated on their spouse and slept with their latest co-actor. Further, those who say they hate it are usually the ones starting it. It's just not worth the stress. One of my best friends, whom I love to death, preaches he hates it, but is so wrapped up in Dramaville that I don't think he'd know how to live without it.

I, on the other hand, can honestly say I loathe it and try everything to stay away from anything drama related. I decided years ago that I wasn't going to be a part of drama's little game and began distancing myself from Jerry Springer-related issues. No soap opera in my life!

After a bit, I noticed an interesting side effect beyond my increased peace. Because I wasn't playing the game, people stopped trying to pull me in. They knew I didn't care, and it wasn't worth their time to convince me otherwise.

Today's Action

Lose drama! Don't read about anything happening to anyone, don't gossip, and if someone tries to tell you what Suzie did, don't let them. Go one day not caring that a co-worker's daughter is now pregnant with her sixth child by yet another baby daddy. You may find it hard, you may feel like you're missing out, but you may discover a whole new side of you that enjoys dealing with your own life rather than the lives of others.

Reflection Time:

- How difficult was it to remove yourself for a day from drama?
- What did you discover about yourself in doing this?

No Solutions

I'm a problem-solver, so it's ingrained in me to find solutions to any issue brought my way. The problem is that sometimes; people need to figure out things on their own rather than rely on others to solve issues. How do we ever learn if we don't make mistakes?

For me, especially as a parent, this is exceptionally difficult. I want to fix everything for my kids, and I've recently learned that sometimes, I just can't. I've also learned that merely being a sounding board can be more effective than being a problem-solver. Allowing someone talk about and work through a situation with you listening can often lead them to discovering answers without you saying a word.

Today's Action:

Today, you're not a problem solver for others. You don't have the answers to anything. You're a sounding board and a great listener. You can guide with open-ended questions, but you can't give answers or advice. This is an exercise for others on self-reliance and an exercise for you on patience.

Reflection Time:

- How did it feel not being able to give answers today?
- What did you find difficult about letting others solve their own problems?

Dress How You Feel

I am probably one of the few proud people on the planet with a zebra-striped cowboy hat. It probably also wouldn't surprise you that I tend to dress a little more boldly than most. See, I dress according to my mood and what I *want* to wear -- not what social norms say I should wear. I try to channel my inner six-year-old who wants to wear the princess dress with the cowboy boots and the red and white Seuss hat to school.

In my corporate position, I constantly struggled balancing what was deemed "acceptable" and my own personal style. I would wear outfits that made me feel miserable and I looked absolutely ridiculous. If I never see another flowered dress with a lace collar, it'll be too soon. Ultimately, my entire wardrobe morphed to black. It was easy, functional and I was ready for a funeral at a moment's notice.

When I left the corporate world and began working for myself, the first thing I did was go through my closet and chucked everything that didn't make me feel fabulous. I decided right there that if I didn't feel like a million bucks every time I put it on, it was outta there. I also wasn't going to buy another thing I didn't absolutely love to wear. I wanted to look in the mirror every day and smile at how awesome I looked.

Do I care what others think about my outfits? Nope! If I like it, I'm wearing it!

Now, I do have to add a small disclaimer: if your work requires you to wear a uniform, by all means, wear it. I don't need emails about people losing their jobs. Also, nudity is not looked upon very favorably in public, so unless you want a visit by the police, I would rethink that option.

Today's Action:

You don't have to completely go crazy here, but for today, wear something you feel really good in. It can be as simple as a "Go to hell" hat or those bangles you absolutely love, but they don't go with any particular outfit. Be bold for just a bit. See where it leads you.

Reflection Time:

- How did you feel being bold and wearing what you really wanted to wear?
- How did you feel looking at yourself in the mirror?
- How are you reconsidering your wardrobe?
- Will you make any changes?

Out Of Character

Ask my children and they will lovingly tell you I'm unpredictable.

They never know what I'm going to say or do next. I laugh too much, do insane things, and constantly keep them off their guard. I've been doing things out of character for so long it's become my character. I *rule* this!

Much to your disbelief, I wasn't always this way. I was always the wallflower girl with glasses who was never asked to the dance. I didn't speak up in class and was happy living a relatively introverted life. I can't say that a spontaneous revelation or life-changing moment started my metamorphosis. I just slowly decided to quit being quiet and bust out of my shell.

First, I started conversations with the people behind the register in the checkout lanes at the grocery store. As that became easier, I talked to people in waiting rooms, in line behind me or at gas pumps. Now, I can speak with anyone. I car danced while riding with my teenage children, started riding motorcycles, decided I wanted to drive my own, and even learned how to sew (which doesn't sound like anything out of character unless you know me. I am just not the sewing type of gal.) I decided to write a book, which became three, tried my hat at a garden (epic fail), tried sushi (love it), am attempting some of the crafts on Pinterest that required the use of power tools. I'm thinking about welding as my next venture.

Today's Action:

Do something you've never done before that no one would expect you to do. Leap out of your comfort zone. Make people wonder if you've been body snatched. Take a step away from the wall and into the spotlight.

Reflection Time:

- How much courage did you have to muster up to do what you did?
- How did you feel once you did?

To The End

I don't know about you, but I'm really good at starting projects and really bad at finishing them. It's not that I intend to leave them incomplete, it's just having little time. I get pulled off the project and never circle back to complete. Occasionally, I'll grab one of my five ongoing crochet pieces and do a few lines while watching TV, but the drive to go for the gold and cross that finish line just isn't there.

Even worse, I know myself so well that I'll delay starting projects because I know I won't get them done. There are a couple of rooms in my house that desperately need painting, but I can't stand the thought of existing under drop cloths for weeks on end. It's not that I'm lazy by any means; life just happens. Just when you're on a roll, your cousin calls because he's run out of gas and you're the only person he could reach, or the teacher calls because your son was playing basketball in the gym, took an elbow to the nose and now it doesn't look like it's on his face straight.

Today's Action:

Today, vow to all that is good and holy - you *will* see a project through to completion. No earthquake, tornado, hurricane or zombie apocalypse shall deter you. In fact, the only thing that will stop you is for the earth to open and swallow you whole. Nothing matters except moving that project from the in progress list to the DONE list. Then you get to do the happy dance and treat yourself to a Blizzard!

Reflection Time:

- Describe the satisfaction of crossing that project off the list of hints you need to do.
- If you make a list of other projects you need to complete, how could you incorporate completing them into your daily routine?

Don't Freak Out

My son was four when he decided one day to pretend he was Native American. He gathered all his markers and proceeded to color every square inch of his body that wasn't covered by underwear. This made complete sense to him, and looking back on it now, his handiwork was pretty good.

When he came downstairs to show me, I had a decision to make. I could either freak out and turn it into a fiasco, or I could choose to laugh my head off until I almost peed my pants. I chose door number two.

Our lives are full of surprises. Some are wonderful and some, completely shitty. But our reaction is key. We can choose to spend our days making things out to be situations of epic proportions, or we can choose to take things as they come, go with the flow no matter what, and have great days in spite of what life throws at us. It's possible. I also have a very old dog, Lucy, who is now incontinent. If I can remain positive as she's urinating while walking across the living room floor, everything else is a breeze.

Today's Action:

When a curve ball is thrown at your head, squash down your immediate gut reaction to fly off the handle and channel Bobby Knight. Instead, take a breath and realize it's not Armageddon. Take care of it, laugh if you can, and move on. There is no sense in letting mess control you or your mood.

By the way, white toothpaste takes ink and marker off skin like magic!

Reflection Time:

- What surprises came your way today?
- Were you able to look at these from a new perspective and how did that feel?
- What other methods do you think you can incorporate to handle life's fast balls?

You Won't Sell Me

I don't think I ever realized how inundated we are with advertising until we made our trip across South Dakota. If you've never been, let me start by saying that it's spectacular! The wide open spaces are absolutely breathtaking!

One interesting attraction you'll come across--and believe me, you will--is Wall Drug. It's located in Wall, SD off I90 and is surrounded by absolutely nothing. The Badlands (named because nothing exists there) are to the south, and flat expanses as far as the eye can see are to the West, North and East. It's been around since 1931, and back then, business was so bad they decided to put up signs in every direction leading toward Wall advertising free ice water (a rarity in the early 1900's) and one cent coffee.

Normally, you would think a few signs would suffice, but not for Wall Drug. Even today, you can see the signs for the free ice water and five cent coffee (inflation) every mile for 100 miles outside Wall. By the time you arrive, you are completely compelled to stop, whether you want to or not. It puts the best hypnotists to shame. You are also so sick of seeing Wall Drug signs that you'll threaten to tear down the next one you spot with your bare hands. Even now, if I see a car with a Wall Drug bumper sticker I want to shake the person and ask "What were you thinking?"

I did, however, learn a valuable lesson from Wall Drug - the power of advertising. At home, we are bombarded with signs, bumper stickers, commercials, and every other means to get our attention. I didn't really notice this until I was in the middle of the most beautiful country I'd ever seen, yet couldn't sit and enjoy it without seeing a sign every few feet. It made me wonder what I'm not seeing at home.

Today's Action:

No advertising. I'll warn you -- this is going to be extremely difficult. Don't look at billboards or signs, please turn down the radio during commercials, and don't read the bumper stickers on the cars in front of you. Instead, look at the other things around you: trees, beautiful houses, pastures and animals. When you catch yourself drifting back to advertising, pull away. You'll be amazed what you notice.

Reflective Time:

- How hard was it to not look at advertising?
- What did you discover new and what did you learn from doing this?
- How can you keep advertising to a minimum in your life going forward?

Just Noticed

Have you ever driven somewhere and realized you don't remember driving the last few miles because you were on autopilot? This is a condition I call zoned-out-itis.

Our frontal lobes are so full of thoughts that our inner brains have to take over driving to keep us from careening into a ditch because we've checked out.

It never ceases to tickle my husband how I can drive a road every day for twenty years and still notice new things. Our conversations go like this:

"When did that get put there?"

"Oh, about fifteen years ago."

"I've never seen it there before."

"Don't know what to tell ya. It's been there since the kids were little."

I don't like to think that I'm just that unobservant, but I am. But, it is actually nice when I notice something I've never seen before. It's like finding Waldo.

Today's Action:

Move out of zoned-out-itis. As you drive around, consciously look for things you've never noticed before in areas you visit all the time. Take notice that the neighbors put in new shrubs or that the new deli opened up in the shopping mall. See how many things you can find that never caught your eye.

Zoned-out-its *can* be beneficial, however. I didn't discover the donut shop for about two years.

Reflection Time:

- What did you discover when you stepped out of zoned-out-itis?

- How shocked were you to find there were things you hadn't noticed before?
- How did discovering you were going around semi-oblivious make you feel?

Think & Act

"Think and act the way the person you want to become thinks and acts!" This is a quote I've incorporated deeply into my life It's a *fake it till you make it* attitude, which is a great way to actually trick your brain into thinking differently. It's looking at the end and taking action to achieve who you want to be.

My "end" me does yoga every morning, is at her goal weight because she eats healthy, is honest and sincere, has many friends, a successful business, and is able to take the entire family of thirty on a vacation once a year. She's Super Matriarch!

I've set really high standards for myself, so until I'm fully there, I'm eating the elephant bite by bite. I eat how my “end” self would eat, which is helping get to my goal weight. I’ve started stretching every morning in an effort to touch my toes again. I’ve written this book, started my second business career as a publisher and will only deal with those I feel are also honest and sincere. My number of amazing friends is growing and we have, so far, been able to pay for enough condos to take twenty-four family members to Florida for a week.

I’m not there yet, but I will be eventually.

Today’s Action:

Think about the person you want to become. What do you like about them and want to emulate? Choose one trait and decide to be like that for today. If you like their confidence, decide to walk a bit taller and purposeful. It doesn't have to be drastic, just one baby step. Remember, "It doesn't take courage to take one step."

Reflection Time:

- What are the characteristics of the person you want to become?
- How did you feel moving one step closer to the person you want to become?
- List the steps you would like to take to make this metamorphosis.
- How can you make daily changes to move you closer?

Trust The Unknown

When I left my corporate job of twenty years, I stepped into the unknown. I knew what I ultimately wanted, but my plan to get there was sketchy at best. I wanted a change, and I would be alright no matter what happened. I looked into the unknown and embraced the hell out of it.

Our gut instinct is to run from things we don't know or understand. This goes back to Caveman Survival 101. The unknown is scary and mysterious, but imagine what life would be like if we knew the outcome of every situation and every action. Sure, we might be safer, but we'd never feel excited about a new venture or grow from our mistakes. This excitement is part of what life is all about. Is it scary? You bet! Do we cave and let fear stop us? Not a chance!

Today's Action:

Step boldly into the unknown. Find something you're shying away from and go for it. Overcome fear and trust that things will ultimately work out for the best. I find trust to be a difficult thing for some because it requires releasing control to the universe. Think of it this way: I'm here to learn from my experiences. My life has encountered both good and bad. If things don't go the way I would like, I can handle it.

Reflection Time:

- How did you take a step into the unknown?
- How did it feel taking that first step and how did it feel once you got over the initial reaction?
- What other ways can you step boldly into the unknown?

Feel The Energy

Reality:

- You are not solid.
- Your body is made up of atoms which have space between them, as well as the protons, electrons and neutrons making up the atom.
- These atomic particles are pure energy, meaning you are pure energy.
- Everything in the world is made up of atoms and energy.
- Your brain also emits electronic impulses as neurons fire, creating thought.
- The law of attraction states that like attracts like. So, negative attracts negative and positive attracts positive.

Based on these, it can be surmised that if you think positive thoughts and emit positive energy, positive energy will be attracted to you. The same goes for negative. Therefore, if you want to change the energy around you, you need to start by changing your thinking.

Today's Action:

First, do the following:

1. Hold your hands in front of you, palms facing each other, but not touching.
2. Move your palms together slowly until you feel something happening between them. It can be heat, a coolness, tingling or they can even feel like they are repelling each other, like magnets. This is your body's energy.
3. You can also hold your palm over your opposite forearm, not touching, and get a similar effect. (This is a great game to play at parties.)

Now that you've felt the energy, think about whether your thoughts are positive or negative through the day. Are you attracting positive or negative things in your life? What type of interactions are you having with others, and can this be linked to your thoughts? Change your way of thinking and see what changes this makes.

Reflection Time:

- What type of sensation did you get when you placed your palms close together?
- How do you think the law of attraction has worked in your life?
- What positive thoughts can you incorporate daily to make sure you're attracting positive energy?

Power Pose

So what made Wonder Woman such a badass? Was it the lasso? The hair? The way she could slice through a gang of bad guys like butter? Obviously. But it was more than that. The image burned into our brains is of her standing, legs spread, lasso hanging from her belt with hands on her hips daring you to get in her way. That was a power pose!

It's been scientifically proven that putting yourself in a power pose not only raises testosterone levels, but it also decreases cortisol (that awful chemical responsible for the spare tire around your middle). Basically, it turns you into a badass and makes you feel awesome. Studies have also shown that someone doing a two-minute power pose before a job interview is more likely to actually get the job. It spikes confidence levels that much!

Today's Action:

Power pose. You want to think big, making your body take up as much room as possible. You can stand in Wonder Woman pose or hold your hands in the air like you just finished a marathon (you can throw in some fist pumps if you like) or sit in a chair, lean back, put your feet on the desk and clasp your hands behind your head. Anything that takes up space and makes you look larger. Stay in this pose for two minutes and feel the attitude change!

Reflection Time:

- What did you feel like after power posing for two minutes?
- Were you able to incorporate it throughout your day?
- How did others react around you? How did it affect them?

Laugh At Stupidity

I was driving in the fast lane, not speeding, but passing a car going slower than me. I was almost past when a little black car flew up behind me, riding my bumper something fierce. I passed the vehicle and was about to get over into the slow lane when the black car whipped over to zoom passed me on the right. I threw up my hands thinking, "If you'd waited five seconds longer, I'd have been out of the way." He replied by actually rolling down his window, in 30 degree weather no doubt, and began flailing his arm out it telling me I was number one.

I busted out laughing!

I realize most people's reaction would be to take offense, get mad and dream of running him down to spit on his carcass, but I just couldn't go there. To see his arm whipping like that out of the tiny car was just too ridiculous. My first thought was how pathetic he looked. My second thought was that Karma was going to have a field day with him.

Today's Action:

When you see someone doing something stupid that should normally put you into a rage or bad mood, laugh at it. It's amazing how simply laughing at situations changes everything. We take life way too seriously sometimes. We're not in a Roman arena fighting for our lives; chill out and enjoy others acting like children. It's rather comical when you stop to watch them.

Reflection Time:

- How did you feel by laughing at situations instead of reacting negatively to them?
- How did doing this all day affect your mood?

Get Up

I've been doing a ton of reading lately about successful people and their habits. I figure that instead of trying to reinvent the wheel, I'd learn from those who have already done it. One common thread I keep seeing is in morning routines. Successful people get up earlier and have more done by 7 a.m. than I have in most of my entire days.

Since I'm not morning material, this practice didn't hold a huge amount of appeal. What I discovered, though, was that when I got up earlier with a plan for my morning, I was so productive. Even better, I carried it with me through the day.

Of course, I was ready for bed by 7 p.m., but I was so productive it didn't matter. Now that I've gotten older, my regular bedtime is 9 p.m. anyway.

The trick to doing this is knowing what you are going to do instead of just shuffling around aimlessly. I go to bed telling myself over and over that I will get up when the alarm clock rings, awake and refreshed. Then I go through what I'm planning to accomplish. For example: I'll tell myself I'll have breakfast done by 5:30. Then, from 5:30 – 6, I'll do yoga. At 6, I'll take a shower and be dressed and ready to go by 7. For some reason, having it all laid out makes me want to get up and get going instead of hitting the snooze button repeatedly. It's tricking my brain into feeling guilty if I don't stay on schedule.

Today's Action:

Tonight, you're going to bed just a little bit earlier so you can get up a little earlier tomorrow morning. You're going to plan out what you're going to do when you get up, and you're going to tell yourself over and over, before you go to sleep, that you will wake feeling refreshed and ready to go. This can be done for even morning zombies like me. You can do this!

<u>Reflection Time</u>:

- What were you able to accomplish by getting up earlier?
- How did it feel to be able to routine your morning?
- How do you think you would benefit from this doing it each morning?

Final Thoughts:

Over the last ninety days, I've asked you to do things that were easy, hard, thoughtful, kind, fun and pushed you out of your comfort zone. In looking back over the journey, I invite you to think on the following:

- What was your favorite day?
- What action was most challenging?
- What actions did you absolutely hate and never plan to do again? Why?
- What three to five actions have you now turned into habits?
- What were the reactions of others as you went through these actions?
- What surprises did you find out about yourself?
- What was one thing you learned about yourself?

- How can you continue to experiment and do something different each day?

I've heard life compared to a rollercoaster. There are ups and downs. Sometimes you laugh. Sometimes you scream. Sometimes your stomach flips and twists inside out until you feel like you're going to throw up. In the end, however, it's a thrilling ride and one you hope to share with those you love.

May you always find peace, beauty, happiness and love!

Sonia

Bibliography

1. Freeman, Jonathan B., et all. *The Journal of Neuroscience.* "Amygdala Responsivity to High-Level Social Information from Unseen Faces". <http://psych.nyu.edu/freemanlab/pubs/2014Freeman_JNeuro.pd>. accessed 6 August 2014.
2. Emmons RA, et al. "Counting Blessings Versus Burdens: An Experimental Investigation of Gratitude and Subjective Well-Being in Daily Life". *Journal of Personality and Social Psychology* (Feb. 2003): Vol. 84, No. 2, pp. 377–89.
3. Ravenscraft, Eric. "Does Speeding Really Get You There Any Faster?" Lifehacker.com. http://lifehacker.com/does-speeding-really-get-you-there-any-faster-1556767685. accessed January 4, 2016
4. Bratman, Gregory et al. *Proceedings of the National Academy of Science of the United States of America.* Nature experience reduces rumination of subgenual prefrontal cortex activation". May 28, 2015. Vol 112 no.28.
5. Jen Sincero. *You Are A Badass* (Running Press, 2013). 164

About The Author

Sonia lives in Lawrenceburg, KY with her husband of 24 years, who she still finds irresistible. They have two sons, one daughter-in-law, and an incredible family of nieces, nephews, great nieces and nephews, in-laws and out-laws.

Her hobbies are reading (of course), crochet, sewing, coming up with new and ridiculous craft projects from Pinterest, riding her motorcycle, and spending time with family and friends. Most nights she's curled up in bed, surrounded by her five dogs, pecking away on her keyboard while *Priest* or *The Strain* plays on the TV in the background.

Her latest literary endeavors may be followed at www.soniagoforth.com or on Facebook at www.facebook.com/soniagoforthauthor. She would love to hear how *For Only One Day* has made an impact in your life.

Bulk Purchase Information

For bulk pricing on purchases of *For Only One Day,* please contact Sonia at soniagoforth@gmail.com.

www.ingramcontent.com/pod-product-compliance
Lightning Source LLC
Chambersburg PA
CBHW030107070426
42448CB00036B/319
* 9 7 8 0 9 9 7 2 2 4 2 0 7 *